Dedicated to my wife Helga,
in love and gratitude,
for her support
and tireless patience.

Dr Bodo Koehler, MD

# Cancer -
# a curable disease

2$^{nd}$ edition 2021-2

Printed and publishing:
BoD - Books on Demand, Norderstedt

**ISBN** 9783754321805

# Preface

There have been myths surrounding the topic of CANCER for centuries. Many books and more studies have been published. Some even with promises of healing. Despite all efforts, this disease is still part of everyday life, and the trend is increasing.

It is noticeable, however, that two thirds of all deaths are still due to cardiovascular disease and cancer only accounts for the remaining 30%. However, the diagnosis of "cancer" is immediately frightening and associated with suffering. Strokes or heart attacks, however, take a back seat.

Where does this polarization come from? Forming opinions is the task of the media. Only bad news can be marketed well. But there are also strong economic interests. There is nowhere near as much money to be made from drugs for the consequences of heart attacks as from cancer and fear. Chemotherapy, for example, is now standard, although only a small percentage of those affected benefit from it. The newer cancer drugs generate even more money if the benefit is dubious. Can it therefore be wanted that one day cancer research will make a breakthrough and that this disease will be defeated?

If there is really interest in a real cancer cure, a systematic review of all research results from the last 150 years would have to be carried out first. The difference to today's scientific work is striking. Due to the lack of high-tech equipment, the work was extremely meticulous and precise. Cheating, as it unfortunately happens again and again today, would have been noticed immediately. In the past there were outstanding personalities who published their knowledge, but who are wrongly forgotten today. Fortunately, transcripts of their work still exist.

I will come back to this in the individual chapters. This book can therefore also be understood as a posthumous tribute to these pioneers. Because they laid the foundations for a holistic understanding of this disease much earlier.

It is also shown; however, that cancer is only an increase in a development that we could call "accumulation of information waste", which is also real material deposits.

But that is only the outward sign of insufficient detoxification activity, on all levels. This requires the uninterrupted provision of EIECs (energy information exchange complexes), a combination of electrons and solar photons (bioplasma). This has much to do with healthy (pollution-free!) diet and love of nature.

The ignorance of rituals such as Lent, the lure of industrially manufactured food and the sedentary lifestyle of many people leave deep marks and exacerbate the problem. But illness up to and including cancer is also a reflection of environmental influences – inside and outside. We experience massive previous damage in a very subtle way through global microwave technology, which was developed as a combat weapon and is now primarily used for surveil-lance. The communication possible with this is just a waste product. Since our organism itself communicates in this frequency range, considerable interference is to be expected here. The development of brain tumors through extended cell phone calls has now been scientifically proven.

Cancer development and detoxification capacity are two extremes of one polarity. With increasing overload of the liver and its detoxification systems (e.g. the glutathione system), regeneration processes in the tissue can derail and get out of control. This is often accompanied by recurrent inflammation with lymph congestion. A successful therapy must start here and first restore the free reflux of the lymph.

Unfortunately, quantum mechanics findings find far too little space in cancer research. We create our own reality by focusing our attention. What is meaningful to us is strengthened – also a source of disease. If fear is added, the development is reversed. Instead of regeneration, it comes to a complete derailment, which we call cancer. If it is not possible to reverse this trend reversal, we can only provide palliative support. But every patient has their own individual chance to stop this inwardly turning spiral!

Despite this goal-oriented approach, it does not cure cancer. The multiple loads on the matrix would not have arisen if the nervous system had been intact and controlled by the brain. This has been overlooked so far.

The loss of control by the brain is an important key. If this is overlooked, progression and relapses can be expected.

The author in summer 2021

# Content

# *Introduction*

In 1998 I published my 150-page book "Synergistic Biological Cancer Therapy" in EDITION CO'MED. It has not lost any of its topicality and is still very recommendable (see bibliography). This new book should be seen as a supplement to bring together old, not yet lost knowledge to combine with new scientific knowledge and to show synergies.

Although there are countless types of cancer and no two symptoms are the same, there is a clearly visible common thread: ***The poisoning of the cell environment when control is lost by the brain.*** This prepares the ground for parasites, mostly fungi, which cause additional damage by producing mycotoxins and thereby letting the process become independent. The tumor itself is just the garbage dump, not the cause.

The garbage can be material, mental, or both. Its increasingly condensed mass disrupts normal functional processes and ultimately also ensures that there is no feedback to the brain and loss of control occurs. Actually, it should have long been noticed that tumors develop painlessly.

Then there seems to be no turning back. But appearances are deceptive: ***Cancer is curable***, even at an advanced stage.

The following explanations show the way, step by step. Actually, a lot is and has always been known; only the horse was bridled from behind. Most therapies focused on the tumor, but were surprised that the disease continued after its removal. The decisive role of the surrounding milieu and its control by the brain, both in the development and in a successful, sustainable therapy, is completely underestimated to this day. That is where the fault lies. With these remarks the attempt is finally made to awaken awareness of it.

# 1. The specifics of cancer

Why cancer? In spite of the billions in research into this disease, there is still no light in sight at the end of the tunnel. There are many reasons for this, which have prompted me to bring some holistic thoughts to a hitherto unsolved problem.

Cancer is not just a human disease. Animals, even trees, can get cancer. To date there has been no real explanation for the mechanism by which malignant tumours develop. However, we can assume that the centuries-long search for a cancer cure was unsuccessful only because the current state of scientific knowledge ***prevented*** a ground-breaking discovery!

On the one hand, this means that the level of knowledge is insufficient. It can justifiably be said that textbook knowledge is not only out of date, but that many contexts are completely misrepre-sented. This applies above all to the complex processes of cell metabolism and the provision of energy in the mitochondria. At the same time I claim that the "guardians of the scientific theses", namely the established scientists, consciously prevent progress. Unfortunately, power interests and corruption are also at play here.

Those who wait for a quantum leap in science are unfortunately waiting in vain, because the system is far too sluggish to make leaps. For each subject there are fixed theories that spread like a blanket over reality. This prevents revolutionary upheavals in science from the outset. It is, however, worthwhile to look for contradictions in today's dogmas for precisely this reason.

## 1.1. Cell division

First, let's look at the process of cell division. In order for a tissue to be able to constantly renew and regenerate itself, the used cells must die. To do this, they use (voluntarily and autonomously!) the mechanism of *apoptosis*, programmed cell death. Then the remains are cleared away by macrophages.

What is little known is that the neighbouring cells that remain behind do not divide afterwards. That is completely impossible with a complex structured cell! Without any exception, the new cells are built from scratch from *undifferentiated stem cells*. These migrate from the basement membrane of the blood vessels into the tissue. They are attracted by electrostatic polarity reversal of the archaic direct current system of the nerve sheaths (see R. O. Becker, "Spark of Life").

**Thesis No. 1**: Adult cells do not divide. Every new tissue cell always arises from a stem cell and differentiates itself from the ground up.

The gradual build-up of highly differentiated cells or tissues is reminiscent of embryonic development, in which all stages of human development are also run through again (phylogenesis). It is similar with stem cells. In their differentiation, they too have to go through each phase of this anabolic process from the beginning (ontogenesis). If errors occur, apoptosis occurs.

The reason for this regular, phased course of tissue renewal is obvious: if an adult cell shows any, if only minor, change, this would after the division be carried through into all subsequent generations.

Since a great deal of damage can occur over time, the organism would no longer be viable in a very short time.

This means that the thesis, currently advocated by conventional medicine, of the first mutation in a single cell, which then triggers cancer, is out of the running. At the same time it becomes clear that the development of a cell tumour must take place on the lowest level, the *stem cell*.

### 1.2. Fermentation as a physiological program

It is often claimed that cancer occurs due to a lack of oxygen in the cells which leads to fermentation. Cancer cells occur much more often, simply through intense physical exertion, without a cancerous tumour developing! On the contrary: the archaic emergency program of fermentation is genetically anchored in every cell. It is even consciously switched on during mitosis, since in the absence of oxygen no ROS (destructive oxygen radicals) can form, which could be dangerous for the DNA after its de-spiraling. Therefore, cells that are fermenting do not become cancer cells. Otto Warburg's thesis is shaken here. Not all fermentation is the same as cancer!

**Thesis No. 2:** The emergency program of fermentation (anaerobic glycolysis) is genetically programmed and does not necessarily represent the transition into a cancer cell.

The specific difference between cancer cells and healthy cells consists solely in the fact that the healthy cell can switch *back and forth* between fermentation and aerobic energy production, but the cancer cell can no longer. It is *unable to regulate* and gets stuck in the fermentation. The mitochondria are switched off in cancer and will remain so. This is how a cancer cell can be defined. However, apoptosis assumes normal mitochondrial function.

What was stated above for the renewal of tissue cells also applies to cancer. Adult cancer cells can no longer divide. Like normal cells, every cancer cell is made from stem cells. Only a *less differentiated cell* can still divide. This is why these cancers are so aggressive.

The further the differentiation has progressed, the more errors occur in the division, which can be observed very well in the microscope. Here, polymorphic, also multinucleated cell formations (syncytium) appear. At this stage, the malignancy is already subsiding because the division rate is clearly declining and approaching zero. Such a pathologically changed cell runs into a self-limiting process with its division. From this it can be deduced:

**Thesis no. 3:** The more clearly the characteristics of a tumour cell (polymorphism, syncytium, differences in colour, etc.), the more harmless the tumour (has become).

Highly *dangerous cells* are *stem cells* that have already become cancerous (see definition above), which leave the original tissue very early and can spread disseminated in the organism. These are even detectable in the bone marrow (by biopsy), which can be demonstrated using the example of breast cancer. It is they who cause recurrences because they have retained their full ability to divide and are only waiting for favourable environmental conditions. You evade imaging procedures completely.

## 1.3. Anabolic strategy

At this point, a first therapeutic approach emerges: Cell division is a catabolic process that is controlled by cortisol and thyroxine. However, only the primitive *stem cells* or poorly differentiated cells can divide.

The *anabolic process of differentiation* must therefore be supported both prophylactically and curatively, or all obstacles must be avoided. The HGH (growth hormone) is primarily responsible for the anabolic side of cell metabolism. For example, it cannot be released in the case of long-term psychological stress (fear !), carbohydrate abuse, and dysregulation of the catabolic hormones cortisol and thyroxine, which are also necessary for cell metabolism, together with the HGH (Fig. 1, Dynamic Balancing of Life).

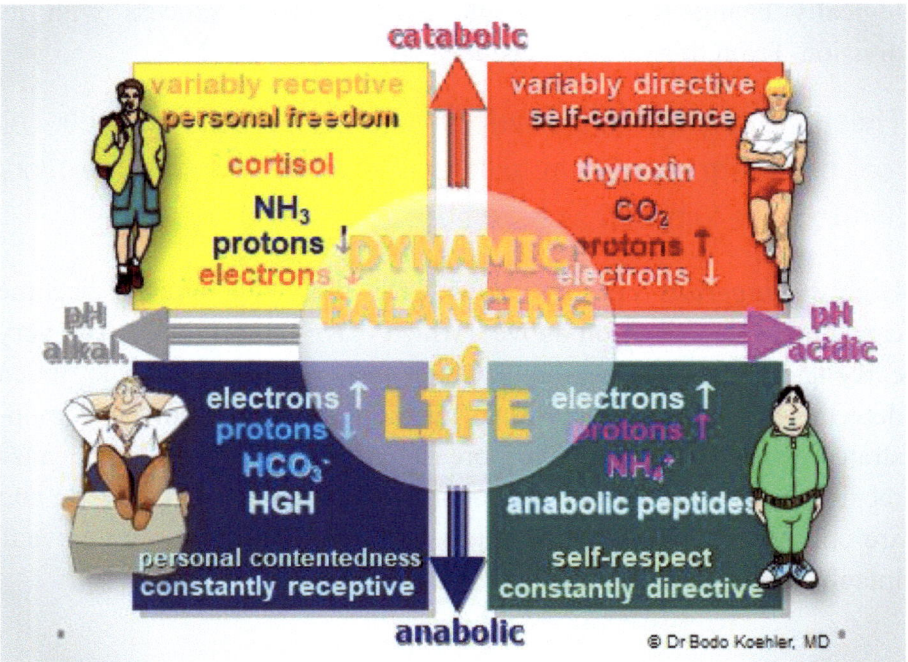

**Fig.1:** Bipolar control of cell metabolism and acids-bases

16

**Thesis No. 4:** The catabolic process of cell division is stopped by increased anabolic activity (differentiation).

### 1.3.1. Oxygen consumption

However, growth processes are associated with an increased consumption of oxygen. In order for enough of it to reach the tissues, oxygen suction is necessary, which is triggered by the ***auto-oxidation*** (self-burning) of certain substances. Above all, unsaturated fatty acids are capable of this, but also certain amino acids such as cysteine. Sunlight intensifies this effect, which is well known from oils in the kitchen, which are therefore kept away from light.

A prerequisite for anabolic processes, which not only include the full maturation of young stem cells, but also every inflammatory and healing process, is therefore a sufficient amount of omega fatty acids (electron donors), ideally in combination with sulfhydryl groups (sulphur-hydrogen in the protein). This is given in the *Johanna Budwig **oil-protein diet.***

Hydrogen bridges (mesomeric bonds) form between the SH groups from the protein and the unsaturated oils, on which the free electrons (so-called $\pi$-electrons) form an electron gas in large numbers. This creates a field effect (through the resonance with the sun), which also affects the solar photons. These are good resonance conditions for red light, which is absorbed by the cells and charges them.

***Oxygen uptake and utilization***, i.e. internal respiration in the mitochondria, is governed by these principles of auto-oxidation. It correlates with anabolism (growth) – regardless of the oxygen partial pressure! This is so remarkable because a person with shortness of breath does not receive any relief from the administration of oxygen (as is routine today) – on the contrary! The situation can even worsen (according to research by Prof Dr *von Helmholtz*), which is regularly shown in the intensive care units, but is not understood. Just a teaspoon of (good) linseed oil will improve the condition in a few minutes. We owe these positive experiences to the fat researcher Dr *Johanna Budwig*. At this point the question may be asked why this basic knowledge has not long since been part of the curriculum.

In her book "Being Human" (MENSCH SEIN) she writes literally:
"All membranes are built up from the partnership between the easily movable electron systems (built from the sun's energy with its electromagnetic fields) and the representatives of hard matter, the sulphur-hydrogen groups in the protein."
And further:
"This love between the electrons of the highly unsaturated fatty acids and the sulphur-containing hydrogen carriers governs the entire metabolism in humans in its flexibility."

In cancer there is little or no oxygen utilization. The growth processes controlled by light and life fail. $\pi$-electrons and the Energy-Information-Exchange-Complexes (**EIEC**s) formed with the photons are the ***anti-entropy factors*** of life. They create order and structure and are responsible for all light absorption in the visible range (all colours).
These connections are absolute and indispensable prerequisites for life!

If the Omega-oils, or the SH-groups, or the sunlight are missing – LIFE is permanently disturbed or even ended in a short time.

It would be nice if we could assume that all people and of course the therapists had been informed about these living conditions for decades and adjusted their diet accordingly by striving for a balanced ratio between omega oils and protein, combined with a lot of exercise in sun light. Unfortunately, it is also not to be expected that the food industry will provide the necessary food in full. The exact opposite is the case!

### 1.3.2. Effect of trans fats

Hardened fats (e.g. in margarine) and long-life oils (polymerized by steam) are still offered and advertised as "healthy".

Trans fats destroy these sensitive life structures and pave the way for serious illnesses. They are even detectable in the tumour mass!

In order to recognize trans fats in finished products, one has to look closely. They are inconspicuously declared as "emulsifiers", or labelled with E 471, 472 or 475. In addition, the Alzheimer's toxin 4-Hydroxy-nonenal (HNE) is formed in highly heated fats (deep fryer!) which – as the name suggests – promotes dementia.

However, a strict distinction must be made between the artificially produced trans fats and the natural forms that arise when the cow's stomach is ruminated. These include, for example, healthy butter and colostrum, but they are also found in lamb.

This already reveals a solution to the problem of tumour development, since it is primarily about the *stem cells*. The question arises: What *prevents* a virgin, completely unblemished stem cell *from obeying* its genetic code and differentiating into a normal tissue cell or, on the other hand, from going into apoptosis when a programme error occurs? Both are directly related to the above-mentioned destroyed foundations of life!

Later we will see that ***information deficits*** due to isolation also play an important role in the undesirable development. Of course, environmental toxins (dioxin – the neurotoxin has been proven to cause cancer), geopathy and technical radiation (here too there are causal relationships) can be brought into the field. All of this can lead to program errors – but apoptosis cannot take place if the above-mentioned livelihoods are missing or have been destroyed by the consumption of trans fats.

That is the point! Problems can constantly arise with cell structure, solely due to the sometimes extremely high environmental pollution (e-smog). This will be either fixed or the cell says goodbye as a whole. But more and more often it happens (with increasing age) that this anchor of apoptosis can no longer be thrown. This shows how crucial the sensitive interaction of oils, protein and sun is for health and well-being.

### 1.4. Stem cells and their milieu
Stem cells are gelatinous, spongy, watery cells. They are all the same. They can be transplanted into foreign tissue at will, and yet only those cells are created that fit into the respective tissue. As soon as they have migrated into a certain organ and perceived (!) their new environment, they grow up as specific tissue cells. If they are transplanted later, however, they remain true to their origin. Who regulates this? Who determines which part of the DNA should be retrieved in which tissue?

**Thesis no. 5:** Specialisation, but also malignant degeneration, does not originate from the cell, but depends on the surrounding milieu.

It has long been known that the extremely large amount of information required for dynamic life processes can never be stored in the DNA. If, however, up to 100.000 chemical reactions take place in a cell per second (in the *entire organism* it is $10^{18}$ per second), then an extremely high information density is required in all cells, and *at the same time.* No cell can work towards simply in front of itself without synchronization with all other cells.

### 1.5. Quantum reality

There are two important terms in the above sentence: *simultaneously* and *total organism*. If information can be accessed everywhere at the same time, then this presupposes a quantum state that enables *collective coherence*. In short, this means: universal simultaneity, or in other words: timeless non-locality.

This *quantum reality*, which can be found everywhere, applies even more to living systems, since not only form and shape have to be maintained here, but also the dynamic life processes themselves. The DNA can be understood as the piano on which the soul plays according to the notes of the spirit. Errors in the system can of course also be due to a defective piano. As a rule, however, it is the "pianist". This is due to the lack of 'entanglement' of the soul with the spiritual quantum space.

It is postulated by quantum researchers that both most of the DNA (so-called junk DNA) and all stem cells are in the quantum state and thus have access to all necessary life information. If you lose this contact, you will be missing important basic information. These can be individual developmental steps up to differentiation, but also the step to apoptosis. This opens the door to cell degeneration, and that is exactly what makes the difference between cancer and non-cancer.

However, the problem is far from being solved with these findings. The second approach for prophylaxis and therapy is logically the recoupling into the quantum space (entanglement with the mind), or the precaution that there is no disturbance of the quantum state in the first place. But how does one do it?

### 1.5.1. Basic building blocks
The electrons come into play again. We want to pay special attention to these small components of matter.
The French scientist, professor of physics, *J. E. Charon*, caused a sensation in the 1980s with his remarks on immortal electrons. The physicist Dr *Michael Koenig* takes up the topic again in his book "Das Urwort – Die Physik Gottes" (The original word – The physics of God, see bibliography). It is worth taking a closer look at this.

The basic building blocks of the universe are remarkably the neutrinos – tiny "forms of being" without mass, which fly through space at different speeds (including superlight) and penetrate all matter.

Two neutrinos (fermions with half-integer spin) rotating around each other form a photon, a light particle (boson with integer spin). Two photons, in turn, combine to form an electron under suitable resonance conditions (sunlight!). However, this does not result in a bundle of different parts, but in a highly ordered structure. This corresponds to a torus (Fig. 2).

These black or white holes are formed by space curvature effects due to the high energy density of the photons. The difference between black and white is that black holes irrevocably swallow matter, while white ones transform it and spit it out again after passing through the inner funnel. In one direction matter forms, in the other it dissolves again in its spiritual origin ($E = m \times c^2$).

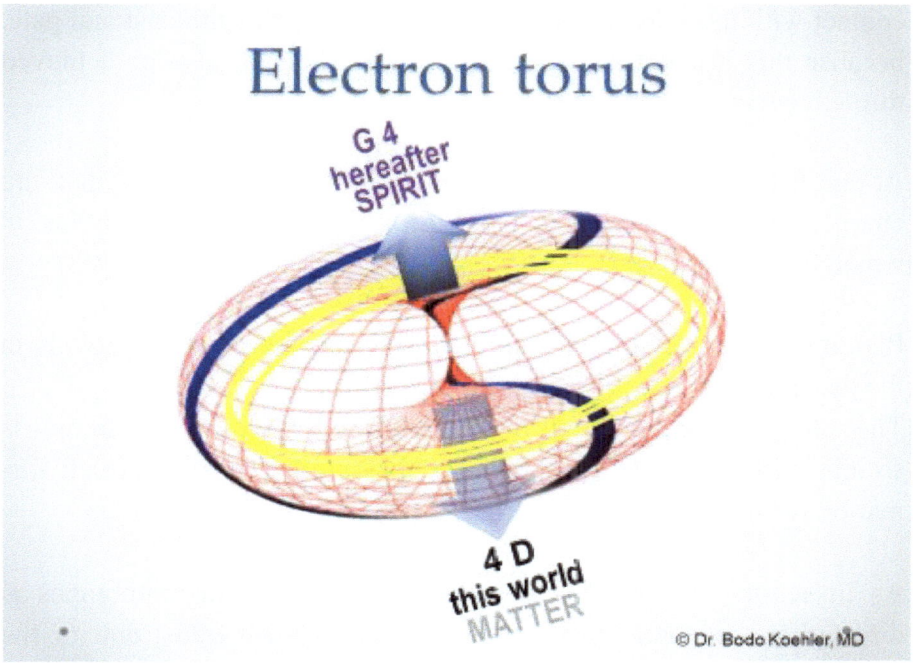

**Fig.2:** The electrons charged with photons are microscopic small black (or white) holes. They are dimensional gates between inner and outer space-time and thus establish the connection between this world and the hereafter. (G 4 stands for hyperspace according to *Burkard Heim*)

The prerequisite for this, however, is that this ring-shaped hollow body is charged with more and more photons that circle around it at the speed of light. But you can also leave it again to exchange ideas with other photons and transfer information (interaction). As a result, the energy level of the electron is raised or lowered again.

In plain language, this means that the more photons have accumulated in the electrons in a loving (!) combination, the easier it is to make contact with the spiritual world beyond through this dimensional gate, because this has increased the coherence. This can also be achieved through concentration in prayer.

A parallel world is formed by *positrons* (anti-electrons) that are charged with anti-photons. This anti-matter forms black holes in which matter disappears.

Photons are usually directed forward into the future; Anti-photons in the past and thus have a destructive effect.

The electromagnetic field of the sun (effective in electrons) is structure-forming, i.e. a prerequisite for auto-oxidation and cell formation (arrow pointing down in Fig. 2).

As in semiconductors, the exchange of electrons in membranes is directed by magnetic fields. Electrons repel each other due to the negative charge, but not if the stored photons contain different information. That makes them attractive. The electrons only repel each other after they have exchanged their information, when they have the same level of knowledge.

So we are already dealing with processes of consciousness at this level. The quantum physics Prof *David Bohm* puts it this way: "The electron observes the environment as far as it reacts to a meaning in its environment. It acts just like humans."

Electrons create an order pull and thus ensure a high quality tissue. However, this is permanently disrupted by technical radiation, especially global mobile communications.

### 1.5.2. Anti-entropy factors

The photons are charged with information from their previous life experience. That makes them intelligent. So you have the knowledge of the past. The further this goes back into the earlier development of mankind and the older you are, the more consciousness is stored. This turns them into so-called *essence electrons.*

These can transfer their long-term experience to other electrons via resonance. So the knowledge is always passed on. This is an act of love that can continue in other people and thus creates a deep connection. This explains why couples can look more and more alike the longer they are connected in love.

These elementary electron-photon complexes can be understood as the smallest units of consciousness.

They are also called **EIECs** (Energy-Information-Exchange-Complexes) because they are responsible for the control of all metabolic processes. They thus form the scientific basis for the *bioplasma*, the often ridiculed "life energy" – the CHI.

A strong electromagnetic field keeps these complex electrons in an excited state. This is one of the positive effects of the sun that cannot be replaced by any "vitamin" D capsule.

But not only harmonic patterns are stored. All injuries are also reflected here. By exchanging the photons, however, a great deal can be automatically neutralized, namely by superimposing positive experiences. This can transform destiny.

**1.5.3. Interference fields** (see Chapter 3.4.4. page 73)
However, if the incisions in life have been too strong and remain unprocessed, i.e. if they far outweigh the positive, then there is a danger of repression. For this purpose, the human being unconsciously builds up a ring-shaped electromagnetic field to encapsulate this area.
Just as a histiocytic wall is erected around an inflammation on a gross level, similar mechanisms become effective on the information level.

This not only binds energy (bioplasma), but also leads to an under-supply of it, which means a lack of light and thus "darkening" in this tissue.

A very large number of people may have had a *violent death* in a previous life. The associated anxiety states can be so severe that they are among the most intensely repressed experiences of all. A large armada of essence electrons is solely concerned with suppressing such events (shield). This significantly weakens vitality and can be the source of seemingly inexplicable, deep-seated fears.
Incorrect dogmatic beliefs, especially in religious questions, can also bind a great deal of bioplasma, which then shows up as an interference field. This can also affect staunch atheists.

At places with reduced bioplasma, "dents" form in the aura, which can be used diagnostically, but also therapeutically, e.g. with balancing therapy (Equalizer EQ 103).

However, if these areas remain unprocessed (as "corpses in the cellar"), it is very easy to see in Fig. 2 that the intellectual information cannot lead to an orderly structure. When passing through the photon ring of the electron, the original information is negatively changed by the contaminated, circling photons, which can produce unnatural shapes.

If we look backwards on this important point of view, it becomes even clearer: The unformed tumour mass suffers from a loss of order and information. So there must have been a distortion (by the transmission of negative information of the photons circling in it) when passing through the electron ring. Since there are innumerable in this encapsulated area, the interference field, this provides a conclusive explanation for the tumour development. It is thus the material image of the stored psych trauma.

A treatment of an interference field is much more comprehensive to be set for this reason than just the elimination of chronic inflammation. It is the interface between psyche and material form, as the basis for possible dysfunction and thus illness – up to and including cancer!

The structure of the tissue is built up by electrons, the shape being given by the stored life information (experience!) in the photons circling in it.

The amazing thing is that *just by remembering and re-engaging* with the subject of injury can these areas be redeemed from the psychic burden. Often this is accompanied by a deep sigh of relief. Talking about it with someone you trust is automatically accompanied by an electron exchange, the unconscious exchange of experience. One person can heal another person completely unconsciously in this way.

### 1.5.4. Primordial fears

However, the *fear of change* plays a very important role here, because the threshold from waking consciousness to the unconscious is controlled by fear! This is therefore a major issue for cancer patients.

The fear centre is known from neuroscience. It sits in the almond kernels (amygdala), which form the anterior tip of the limbic system on both sides. This is significant because there is a material substrate for the symmetry in the controlled action. The emotional right hemisphere should be in balance with the rational left hemisphere. If there is an asymmetry here, i.e. a preponderance of anxiety-producing thoughts, then careful, considered action becomes stressful action, even panic, with greatly increased energy consumption, which can lead to catabolic derailment.

This not only leads to an increased consumption of bioplasma, but also stresses the kidneys (blue quadrant Fig. 1), which are responsible for basic trust and calming the system. High blood pressure is therefore a pioneering symptom that should not simply be suppressed with medication.

It should not go unmentioned that the new 5G mobile radio standard, due to its short wavelength, directly resonates with the amygdala, which is only a few millimetres in size, and can thus trigger unconscious fears. Wrong decisions are made under fear, which opens the door wide to any kind of manipulation.

We are now very close to solving the cancer problem. So if we have the courage to (re) deal with the old repressed issues, especially those that are associated with fears of death, bioplasma can flow again and the "dents" can be compensated, which brings health closer.

And what about the deposited trans fats? With enrichment of the bioplasma, intensive detoxification can be carried out again and the deposits can be removed. That would actually be all done.

That sounds good, but is only suitable for prophylaxis!
The difference to the patient already suffering from cancer is serious. The longer the double load goes, due to deposits in the matrix on the one hand and the interference field with a lack of bioplasma on the other, the faster the nervous system degenerates in this area, which leads to a loss of control by the brain. The further process is thus irrevocably determined. The process has now reached a full degree of autonomy that cannot be reversed by it.

In my decades of work as a doctor, I have repeatedly asked myself desperately why after intensive therapy and changing all stressful factors in lifestyle, turning to new tasks and returning joy in life, in some cases the tumour came back, often worse than at the beginning.
Here is the clear answer: The mental demands are transmitted to the tissue via the nervous and hormonal systems, and from there feedback is sent to the brain. This is especially the case with inflammation. All healing processes are controlled and monitored from the brain.

However, if there is massive previous damage on site due to deposits, loss of bioplasma with difficult oxygen uptake and utilization, loss of information and the formation of a tissue 'lump" – the tumour that corresponds to the stressful psychological topic, no therapy or other measure is sufficient if it is not possible to re-create the above-mentioned life conditions in the tissue.
For this reason, many different possibilities on this therapeutic path are discussed in later chapters, because treatment can only be carried out individually so that the desired success is achieved.

What is not needed is dismantled. It is a law. This not only affects muscles and bones (e.g. after a bone break), but all organs, especially the nervous system. Disused areas, and these are the interference fields, are also part of it. To make matters worse, there are many neurotoxic viruses on the way that accelerate the breakdown or trigger it in the first place. These include, for example, chickenpox, which can break out again in old age as herpes zoster (shingles).

Unfortunately, vaccinations can also do this if they encounter a weakened or not yet fully developed immune system (infants!). Then the trigger is set very early.

The indispensable stimulation of the formation of new nerves (neuro-neogenesis) is understandably particularly difficult, but it is indispensable. We expect healing only when the organism can function again as a unit, as a whole (collective coherence).

## 1.6. Ontogenesis

First of all, reference must be made again to the developmental steps of the embryo and the stem cells until they are fully developed. The reason for these growth stages lies in the "operating instructions". It would make little sense and would only wreak havoc if the entire blueprint were implemented from the start. The *exact sequence* of the construction steps is more important than the overall information. Just by confusing the order (with otherwise complete information content) chaos would arise.

In the case of a house, the roof cannot be put on before the walls have been erected. If you set priorities here, the correct order seems to be even more important than the overall content, because improvisations may be allowed there. This is where the *nervous system* comes into play, in two ways (see later).

"Sequence" means sequence of events that must first be brought to full maturity individually.

This law applies to all areas, regardless of whether it is the development of humans from embryo to adult or individual cells (ontogenesis). Errors in the later structure and thus the function can be traced back to an incorrect development step. This is of course in the past and is therefore tied to a certain time – but also to the respective event!

Structural errors correspond to non-transformed time events!

If the "structure" is a tumour, it would be imperative to seek out the stressful event in the past and transform it afterwards. This is not only possible, it would be causal therapy!
However, one always has to consider what soil an agent hits. The condition of the *entire organism* is decisive for the effect.

If we keep in mind that animals and trees can also get cancer, then a common principle must be effective. It is now certain that *geopathic disorders* have a cancer-promoting effect on all living systems. The type of field disturbance has not yet been researched, which proves that it must be an "imprint" in the universal quantum space. If the cause of the disturbance were measurable, it would no longer be in the quantum state.

## 1.7. Organizational fields
Scalar fields are not static, but rotate, not just in one direction, but at the same time opposite polarity, whereby they neutralize each other. This prevents their measurability.

There are several types of fields. Due to their dynamics, they can transform into one another through induction, e.g. an electric field into a magnetic field and vice versa.

The ones known today are – besides the ones just mentioned – the gravitational fields and the scalar fields. Other subdivisions are morphogenetic field, subquantum field, quantum field, potential field, etc. Further fields that are still unknown today have to be postulated. The home of all fields is the vacuum or zero point field, i.e. the spirit.

The maser hologram of the neural network, which is described in detail in chapter 4.5., has a special significance as a comprehensive field.

## 1.8. Alkalosis

A stem cell gets the impulse for the division from its direct environment, but not the DNA. The stimulus to divide always comes from the environment, where more and more cell death occurs, e.g. as part of a recurrent inflammation.

However, division only ever takes place under *alkaline conditions*. The stronger the alkalosis, the faster the division. That is why all regeneration processes mainly take place at night in an alkaline environment. The normal pH value in the tissue is 7.0 to a maximum of 7.1, so it only becomes slightly alkaline at night. Everything above it is pathological and can stimulate normal cell division in such a way that loss of order is favoured.

Who or what is actually responsible for the pH value in the tissue? Who controls the acid-base balance?

These are essential questions that are rarely asked. The rough control takes place in the organism via the polarity of carbonic acid (or $CO_2$) and bicarbonate (compare Fig.1 page 16). The fine regulation, however, which takes place mainly on the membranes, is due to the $\pi$-electrons in the unsaturated fatty acids (have a deacidifying effect), together with the hydrogen groups of the proteins (have an acidifying effect).

However, the cell is not passively dependent on the environment. Its reaction is the active response (adaptation) to its environment. The milieu sets the living conditions for the cells. It is also the environment that can drive a cell into degeneration.
It suddenly becomes clear why there can be so many and varied carcinogens. They change the environment by drastically reducing the number of free electrons and, at the same time, the number of protons. (cancer cells remains alkaline for life!). On the one hand radicals are capable of this, on the other hand all alkalizing substances, especially alkaloids (fungal poisons), which also have a neurotoxic effect (Chap. 3.2.1.1. page 65).

This can also be done indirectly, for example by stimulating the production of one of the strongest cell poisons and alkalizers at the same time: *ammonia*. This gas is produced in all putrefaction processes, especially in the intestine, puts a massive strain on the liver and must actually be regarded as the most important co-carcinogen, because it penetrates all tissues, even the brain.

This is another factor in the risk of cell degeneration: tissue alkalosis increases the speed of division extremely, which means that errors can occur more frequently in the complex division process. Because the increased stimulus to division also affects those cells that have already started to differentiate, which is not the case under *slightly* alkaline conditions. This increases the error rate. This becomes particularly dangerous when it hits the programmed mechanism of apoptosis.

But there is still a braking mechanism, and that is the free electrons. In the so-called reducing milieu (blue and green quadrants in Fig. 1, page 16), degeneration is virtually impossible. It was only in the substantial absence of electrons (from the unsaturated fatty acids), but also of protons (yellow quadrant) can arise cancer.

### 1.9. Consciousness

"Information strives for meaning" (says quantum physicist Prof *Th. Goernitz*). This means that the spiritual content of an idea (information) can only be realized when it materializes. But giving meaning is reserved for mind-driven living systems.

So apparently the purpose of life is to act as a testing platform for the spirit, a tool so to speak. If a person integrates this fundamental aspect into his or her thinking, then suddenly there is a deeper meaning for every situation in life, including cancer. At this moment affected patients can see why they are sick and how they can get out of it. This is a good prerequisite for healing.

Spirit recognizes itself in the *form*. In human, he recognizes his *work*.

A formless structure like cancer obviously lacks the meaningful information of the spirit.

A positive, life-affirming mental and spiritual attitude will most likely contribute to supporting the dynamics of life processes, because life means constant change, means "learning by doing" – learning through implementation (of the needs). This includes an open willingness to face the daily challenges without fear and with great curiosity and joy in the new knowledge gained.

*New entanglement with the quantum space (spirit)* crystallizes out as a golden key, but cannot be generalized and filled into tablets.

Ultimately, "entanglement with quantum space" does not mean anything else than the intense turning to God in **LOVE**.

The great hope for curing cancer, which is actually still possible at any (!) stage, lies in the fact that there is actually a logical development as the background to the development of cancer, which is shown here and which can be reversed. The necessary change in awareness can be initiated by changing the context with a new task.

The implementation of these findings is clearly in the hands of each individual. It is a very promising approach, and it is elaborated further in the following chapters, along with entirely new aspects.

**Findings**

*Important findings are revealed right at the beginning. Adult cells can no longer divide, which would be completely pointless, since one old cell would become two old cells. Although that doesn't make any sense, it's still in the curriculum.*

*Fermentation doesn't mean cancer. It is a physiological process that is used more often than initially assumed, namely with every cell division. To derive a cancer diagnosis from this would be premature.*

*It is also incorrect to infer the malignancy from the sometimes extremely changed cell morphology. The stronger the change, the less growth is possible.*

*Orderly growth (anabolic) goes hand in hand with increased oxygen consumption. Certain requirements are required for this. According to J. Budwig, it is unsaturated fatty acids as electron donors that are charged with information-carrying solar photons – in conjunction with the sulfhydryl groups of certain proteins. This enables auto-oxidation and controls oxygen uptake and processing.*

*If – as is unfortunately the case today – trans fats are constantly consumed, these EIECs collapse and with them gradually all life processes and structures.*

*If the anabolic process of differentiating a stem cell is successfully promoted without any gaps, the development of cancer is ruled out. For this purpose, the laws of regulation of cell metabolism according to Prof Dr Dr Juergen Schole can be used consistently.*

*In the meantime, it should also be understood that the cell should only ever be viewed in conjunction with its environment, because there is a lively exchange of information here. The health or disease of a tissue depends on this alone.*

## 2. Cancer from perspective of Life-Supporting Medicine

Is there a cancer constellation or can it affect everyone? Just as only a certain percentage of people get sick during a flu epidemic, this applies in principle to every illness. Those who do not belong to the risk group are mostly spared. That should actually also apply to cancer. But what specific factors promote the outbreak of this dreaded disease? Is there a so-called "cancer personality"? Or is it the case that cancer is an exception to other dispositions in chronic diseases and cannot be predicted?

### 2.1. The categorical classification system

What we lack for assessing this question and for medicine as a whole is a system of order that allows clear, contradicting statements and at the same time shows the interactions of various aspects. Only then can one work scientifically exactly, instead of relying on statistics that completely negate the main aspect of a person, namely his individuality.

Unfortunately, it is not well known that such a categorical system in the form of the **Luescher cube** (according to the Swiss psychology Prof Dr *Max Luescher*) has existed for over half a century, but has not yet found its way due to the linear-causal system of thought in conventional medicine.

The categorical classification system is compatible with the 5 change phases of TCM (*Taoist* Chinese Medicine), which underlines its universal validity.

Since the Luescher cube has a multi-dimensional and bipolar structure, it not only obeys the geometry of the room (structure, composition, expansion), but also conforms to the ancient teaching of the 4 elements (fire, water, earth, air). As a result, all the influences to which matter is exposed are reflected in it. Since in ancient China only 4 elements were assumed as the basic principles (not 5, as later in traditional Chinese medicine), everything fits together. Due to translation errors, 5 conversion phases became 5 elements. Only through rediscovered old writings could the error be cleared up.

But it is precisely the 5 phases of change that lead us to important insights, especially if they are derived from the Taoist original doctrine of the I-Ching and applied in several dimensions.

"Metal" corresponds to the air element. There, the lungs and large intestine are found as functional groups, as well as grief (loss) and resignation as psychological correlates.

We breathe in PRANA through the lungs, spiritual food according to Ayurveda. Breathing itself is a function of the kidneys (!), which belong to the water element. The large intestine should no longer contain anything undigested, but rather draw water (!) from the digested nutrition. The functional system *metal* (air) lung / large intestine converts the energy and passes it on to the *water element* kidney / bladder, which is why the lungs are also known as the "mother of the kidneys".

These complex relationships between metal (air) and water alone make it easy to imagine disorders of the functional circuit kidney / bladder.

The assignment in the Luescher cube now gives rise to further interesting aspects. The air element (yellow) is variable-receptive and separative (Fig. 3 next page). A cancerous tumour is a prime example of isolation and thus separation.

38

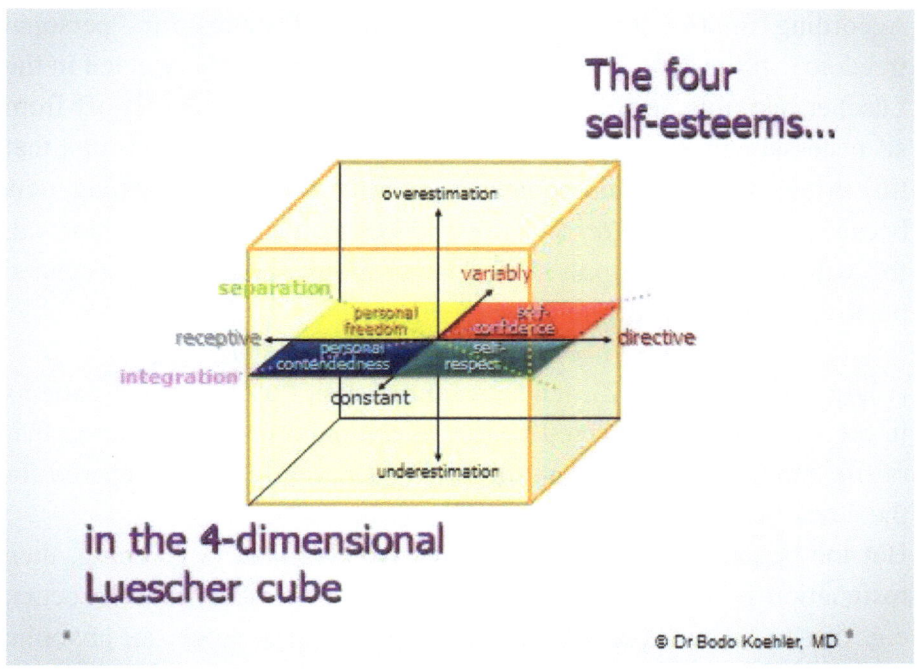

**Fig.3:** The Luescher cube – the categorical classification system
according to the Swiss psychologist Prof Dr *Max Luescher*

The water element is constantly receptive and integrative. Water as a universal solvent connects everything with everything in the organism and thus ensures coherence. Only then does it make it possible for "relationships" to be built up between the individual components and for them to acquire "meaning".

An unwanted separation (loss of relationship) must therefore be countered with re-integration. This is one of the main tasks of the kidney / bladder functional circuit in connection with the functional circuit *heart / small intestine* and *3-E / circulation* (both fire element) and thus also the thyroid gland.

Blue and red form the axis of integration.

According to *Max Luescher*, the air element stands for "personal freedom". If the associated sun yellow is predominantly rejected in the Lüscher test, this person closes himself off and cuts himself off from all necessary renewal processes, but also from new relationships that life brings with it. This equates to a refusal to face anything new because of a *fear of life*. But life and health mean constant renewal, for which external impulses and suggestions serve. The associated positive emotion is "desire for something new".

A large-scale study in Zurich showed that over 80% of cancer patients in the Luescher test rejected yellow as the main colour. With the fear of life and the future in front, the way is apparently being prepared for the development of cancer.

But the beginning is important. If the development is creeping, then resignation is more likely than cancer. But if a sudden event occurs, e.g. due to an unexpected loss, combined with a shock, an anabolic derailment occurs (due to insufficient catabolic activity). The blue-red integration axis is permanently disturbed (red in deficiency), which is immediately perceived as an existence-threatening fear due to the loss of energy (weakens the water element kidneys / bladder).

We do not find the effects on the blue-red integration axis, but at a 90° angle (reciprocally) on the yellow-green separation axis. Since all development processes always have a reciprocal cause, which corresponds to the right angle, it is no longer possible to integrate, it will be separated (see Fig. 1 and 3).

But be careful! There is only a risk of cancer if there is a loss of authenticity on the separation axis in green (self-respect) to *external control*. This means overlaying (interference) with external information from other living beings, up to and including microbes, e.g. fungi (see later).

This imbalance on the separation axis must be corrected on the integration axis, which can lead to excessive demands in the red quadrant (energy supply, heat). This increases the inability to heal inflammation (blue quadrant) in the specified time window (1 week acute + 3 weeks convalescence), which can be considered a pre-cancerous stage.

This shows very nicely that all 4 poles always interact with each other and never one alone. That is why every linear-causal approach to humans is characterized by errors and, especially when assessing chronic diseases, doomed to failure (see Fig. 9, page 78).

Prof *Grossarth-Maticek* (University of Heidelberg) was able to find out another essential aspect of the development of the disease through an extensive survey of cancer patients (and heart attack patients), namely "unmet needs". This leads to years of agonizing ***development backlog*** by renouncing things that one would have liked to live out.

Here, too, there is a rejection of life with untried opportunities and thus a lack of ***new relationships.*** This refusal corresponds to the not lived red (integration axis) and thus the lack of implementation of these suppressed wishes. The positive effect would have been a strengthening of self-respect (green), which grows through experience.

But it's not just about the big things in life, but also and above all about the many small needs that show up on every level – from the cells to the entire organism. The individual systems always strive for balance because this saves energy. Deficiencies can prevent this, as can information deficits.

41

The study from Heidelberg, which was carried out over 20 years, also proved that the foundations for problems in life are laid in childhood, primarily through conflicts between children and her parents. Here the *feeling of deep security*, usually conveyed by the mother, plays the decisive role.

Every rejection, every longer absence, e.g. due to illness, or the loss of the mother for other reasons has serious consequences for later life.

In this context, shamans report the consequences of a violent death in previous lives, which could very well explain the urgent need for closeness and security, but above all love. Because behind this there is of course a deep-seated, mostly completely unconscious fear. This activates the amygdala (on both sides at the front tip of the limbic system) and puts it under constant stress. In this context it is interesting that in autistic people a clear enlargement of this fear centre can be determined. They are known to lack the ability to align their actions with feelings, which can lead to uncontrolled actions.

Equally important is the fact that microwave radiation from mobile radio, especially 5G (!), Due to the short wavelength, resonates with the two amygdala centres. This influence on the fear centre has a direct effect on the kidneys, the seat of life energy from the point of view of TCM.

This "ancient" idea has long since been underpinned by biophysics. The "life energy" or the Chi of the ancient Chinese is called BIOPLASMA in science. It consists of innumerable electrons that are charged with information-carrying photons, i.e. light quanta (see Chapter 1.5.1.).

Using the example of breast cancer, the development of cancer can be well understood on a psychological level.

## Breast cancer genesis according to Prof Grossarth-Maticek

- Almost always massive rejection / separation experience from the mother
  Breaking a continuous, mutually loving and appreciative relationship

- Attempting the repair in adulthood with another person
  Long-term hope for love and attention (++ 1, brackets)

- After another disappointment, all attractive objectives are blocked
  Mental and physical Exhaustion and aggravation of risk factors (diet, inflammation)

- The person cannot experience their role as a woman in an attractive way
  She experiences herself in the disappointed child role (- - 4)

- Balance TO FEEL LIKE <> NOT TO FEEL LIKE shifted to the right

According to his theory, the balance between pleasure and dis-pleasure, but also the denial of pleasure (self-punishment through false feelings of guilt and not lived needs) plays a major role.

Various triggering factors can be seen, which are shown schematically here using several examples. The approach to resolution results from the *autonomy training* he developed.

## Polarities according to Prof Grossarth-Maticek
Specific trigger factors

- Breast cancer: Strong mother bond with constant rejection
Dissolution through the certainty of being deeply loved by the mother in spite of everything

- Testicular cancer: Strong father bond with constant rejection
Dissolution through the certainty of being deeply loved by the father in spite of everything (achievement)

- M. Parkinson's: Intense, chronically uncontrollable fear, fatalism
Resolution of resolving fear-inducing conflict situations (limbic system)

- M. Alzheimer: Listless and stressed displeas. rejection of new suggestions
Dissolution through the targeted search for new opportunities to participate in life

- Heart attack: The feeling of being helplessly exposed to a negative object
Dissolution through the learned ability to distance oneself from the object

All results were determined to be highly significant in the Heidelberg study and are taken from the book "Synergistic Preventive Medicine" (see bibliography).

In testicular cancer, the disturbed father relationship is very strong, but not only there. The father stands for achievement (red quadrant in the Luescher cube) and often puts pressure on the sons (less often daughters). This leads to permanent stress with all negative consequences.

The following assessment of cancer-promoting factors comes from the above book (quote):
"A person strives for an object with the highest level of emotional activity (e.g. closeness to and recognition of a person, a certain achievement of a goal in professional life), but repeatedly experiences that the object is finally no longer attainable. Nevertheless, the person is not able to distance himself from the object, which leads to inner despair, emotional and physical exhaustion, negative experiences, inner hopelessness, etc. This state is usually covered over by adaptation and altruism.
There is an internally encapsulated suffering in isolation, which can no longer be reduced by the behavior or converted into pleasure."
(End of quote)

However, one crucial point must not be overlooked, which was clearly shown in the Heidelberg results: Cancer (like any other disease) is never monocausal, but always the result of *all* interactions to which a person is exposed.
The examples listed here must therefore be related to the context, the physical constitution (e.g. inflammation sources), the lifestyle, etc.

This gives rise to indications, i.e. ***probabilities,*** which must be further supported diagnostically.

If people at risk either have a good ***family and / or work climate***, then several negative influences are compensated for. These two factors apparently play a decisive role, because here the aspect of ***love and affection*** plays a role.

However, if ***fear of an illness*** is in the foreground, the risk can increase by a factor of 10. This was shown in smokers who were afraid of cancer.

Health requires (according to Prof Dr Dr *Juergen Schole*) constant ability to change and adapt, which is not the case under the conditions of a thought carousel.

Another scientist puts it this way:

## Prof Dr Richard Davidson (Neuroscientist University of Wisconsin-Madison)
*4 neural networks* control our well-being:

1. The ability to maintain positive states
   - This requires love and compassion

2. The ability to concentrate and keep negative thinking away
   - Meditation techniques and prayers are helpful for this

3. The ability to be generous
   - This is best learned through caring for others

4. The ability to recover from negative states
   - This requires an open eye for new possibilities

These 4 networks work independently of each other. The individual points correspond to the 4 quadrants in the Luescher cube. Each of them not only shows possible disorders, but is also a causal approach to therapy.

According to Prof *Franz Ruppert*, the basic need of every human being is *to live, to love and to be loved.*

At this level it's always about the whole. At the moment when blind, destructive hatred turns into deep love (e.g. against parents or partners), spontaneous healings are tangible.

## 2.2. Collective coherence

Another aspect must not be overlooked, even if it is not yet scientifically common knowledge: Life is unimaginable if we did not consist of *highly intelligent*, *self-regulating cells*, due to the close interweaving of our controlling soul with the material structures of ours body. The cells see themselves as an integral part of the community of the cell state and submit to our will. This enables *collective coherence*. This intelligence is an expression of the entanglement with the quantum space (spirit), from which all life processes are controlled, whereby the DNA (cavity resonator) has the function of an information converter.

Creating *relationships* to try out *possibilities* that are selected from the immeasurable potential of the quantum field (zero point field, spirit) via *emotions* is one of the basic requirements for life.

## 2.3. Thoughts quantum field

All events have their origin in the quantum field (spirit), but all experiences made with them are also stored there (see morphogenetic field according to R. Sheldrake). Nothing is forgotten, nothing is lost.

As in Chap. 1.5.1. executed, the light quanta circling in the photon rings provide universal storage for all previous, but also much earlier events and experiences.

This fact is significant because the force of events caused many cancer patients at some point to decide to die. If this death information is not actively transformed later, it continues to have an uninterrupted effect, even if this person has long since rearranged himself, settled in again and long ago forgotten the event. At that time the entanglement with the original information in quantum space was "contaminated" by stressful thought constructs (compare Fig. 2 page 23).

Well-being and satisfaction are no indications that a time bomb is not slumbering deep down. It is not uncommon for this to be shown in the Lüscher test many years later. But regardless of this, it can be postulated that such an unprocessed event with a *longing for death* is stored in very many cancer patients.

According to Dutch authors, these are split-off parts of the personality (as disturbance fields) that develop their own dynamics as entities (egregore), right up to their materialization as a tumour. This corresponds to the view of the shamans, who unfortunately are wrongly denied recognition as "medicine men".

"Cancer is nothing more than a materialized thoughts quantum field structure." Prof Dr Jules Muheim

In the kinesiological test, this unconscious stress can lead to the result that the affected patient would rather (not knowingly) be sick rather than get well. An intensive discussion is necessary here.

The already mentioned Heidelberg sociologist Prof *R. Grosshardt-Maticek* writes in his book "Synergetic Preventive Medicine" Chapter 7 on page 50 verbatim (beginning of the quote):

"The human organism as an extremely complicated system of inter-action develops an enormous number of needs on the different biological, psychological and social levels (e.g. to minimize the constant tension between the actual and the target state).

We assume that the goal of a socio-psychobiological individual is to achieve the *highest level of interactive needs satisfaction (in different systems) leading to pleasure and well-being,* so that ultimately well-being can be experienced. The organism also tries again and again to eliminate or bypass sources which, acutely or in the long term, lead to inhibitions in the satisfaction of needs.

The central nervous system systematically registers sources of dis-pleasure and pleasure and relies in particular on information stored emotionally and cognitively (e.g. in the limbic system). The *pleasure qualities experienced as the highest in the individual life story are activated again and again* (from memory) and an attempt is made to repeat them or to restore them in a similar way (e.g. with similar or similarly associated objects, the originally strong pleasure reactions have caused). Likewise, sources of the greatest displeasure are stored in the memory, whereby an attempt is made here to avoid them in the future.

-   .   -

It is therefore of central importance for problem solving of all kinds in which communication systems people strive for and achieve pleasure, well-being, security and development and in which systems blockages occur." (End of quote, italics according to the original).

Today we know that up to 40% of female breast tumours regress spontaneously without the patients being aware of it and without the appropriate therapy.

From a quantum physics point of view, ignorance is the best way to let things go undone. Because reality only arises when we give *meaning* to the events. A target-oriented strategy can be derived from this, through the following basic law

Faith creates reality – doubt erases it.

Should a cancer diagnosis actually be made one day, it is allowed this by no means immediately believed, but should be immediately called into doubt, because there are actually very many reasons to question such a serious statement. Findings are often incorrect or contradictory. Anyone who is able to decisively reject the topic of cancer – not out of ignorance, but out of deep inner conviction – does not have to get sick, or has the best (spontaneous) chances of recovery!

In such cases, however, a positive milieu change has often taken place without being noticed (external influence warded off!), because the progression of the disease primarily depends on the environmental conditions – inside and outside (context).
Anyone who does not receive support at home or among friends, but continues to be exposed to negative influences that "poison the atmosphere" has only one chance: to break out of their surroundings.

## 2.4. Context
Anyone who has established a relationship with someone or anything, e.g. an important (!) thing, remains connected to this person / thing through the "entanglement" even if a spatial separation has occurred – voluntarily or involuntarily through *loss*. Certain parts of a person

then continue to resonate with the missing "partner" (even beyond death), which is why a loss is experienced as no longer "being healed" or even directly as an external influence and has acquired "meaning".

The missing part has created a sensation of "no longer be complete" and "torn out" a piece of the whole of the human being. This "leak" can be occupied by foreign entities, which is where the real danger lies.

"Leak" means the loss of bioplasma and with it countless positive essence electrons. A picture of two trees standing close together can be used as a comparison. As long as both are well, they form a beautyful, harmonious unit. If one day a tree is missing – whatever – an ugly gap has arisen, on the side of which branches are missing and the imperfection, the "disaster" becomes visible.

A tree can change a lot by producing new shoots at this point and thus compensating for the loss. But what does a person do in a comparable situation? Symbolically, it would be advisable to follow the laws of nature and also to develop new "shoots", to initiate new things, to open for new contacts (yellow aspect). Before that, however, the loss should be neutralized through acceptance, understanding, forgiveness and transformation.

The most important relationship that should be established is with you and at the same time (!) with all of creation; to *feel* part of it. There is a term for this relationship that has unfortunately become too banal – LOVE.

Love is the universal force that holds everything together and thereby enables the necessary unity of an organism in the first place.

This is actually where scientific research should start to find out what kind of energy love actually represents.

With the appropriate expansion of consciousness, every person can compensate for deficits like a tree and return to harmony (= health, to be healed).
But be careful: Compensation should by no means be understood as substitute satisfaction. Only that which is authentic should be consciously built up, nothing foreign should gain access.

Ultimately, a tumour is nothing more than a landfill of unprocessed external influences (see above). This "accumulation" poisons the environment of the cells in the immediate vicinity, as a prerequisite for further tumour spread. Which tissue is affected first is shown in the system of the 5 phases of conversion taking into account the psychological correlate, which closes the circle.

From this point of view, it makes sense to understand cancer as a fall from one's own spiritual destiny, which makes life on earth meaningless.

*In summary*, it can be stated: A person who has a cancer constellation often has the following characteristics:
  ➢ Disturbed mother and / or father relationship
  ➢ Falling out of one's own spiritual destiny
  ➢ Unrecognized purpose and purpose in life
  ➢ Loss of joy in life, with a feeling of inferiority
  ➢ Unlived emotional needs, adapted, externally determined
  ➢ Previous experience of shock due to unexp. loss of relationship
  ➢ Repressed, not withdrawn decision to die
  ➢ Permanent conflict, unwillingness to rethink

> ➤ Lost ability to love, to forgive, to forget
> ➤ External milieu (family, work place) that preserves or strengthens the situation (context)

## 2.5. Importance as an aspect of consciousness

This term can change the sense of life. Only that becomes reality for us to which we attach ***importance***. This term is of almost inconceivable scope. It determines our lives like no other and results from the emotions with which we control our intentions. By giving ***meaning*** to something, reflection creates a standing wave that opens up a timeline. The "thing" thus endures and has become a personal reality.

The first step towards healing is to become aware of these relationships and to understand the indispensable necessity of a transformation in all areas mentioned here.

Only when the patient gives the ***life*** processes the meaning that is necessary for healing and builds new, sustaining relationships in love (not least with him!) can he / she become healthy. It is about the inner cohesion of all (!) components in the sense of a community action ***"life"*** – one for all, all for one, with joy and vigour. Physics calls this coherence.

We can perceive it as a ***sense of community***, which leads to deep security and trust. What is meant here is not only the cohesion of our cells, but also the personal relationship to the whole of creation and to God.

## 2.6. Therapeutic considerations

In **LSM**, the Life-Supporting Medicine, we proceed according to the 3 + 1 law. The main task is to return to the authentic structure by reintegrating the refused, untransformed aspects (conflict congestion), which correspond to the split off tissue part – the tumour. Rejection means deprivation of love!

That is why therapeutically the yellow aspect that is not lived (opening up for new adventures) is strengthened by using the integrative water element (blue aspect), which connects everything, with its diverse properties to help on the tumour area. In this way the balance on the integration axis is restored so that it can do its job properly (compare Fig. 1 und 3). This improves the (disturbed) ability to resonate (love!) with the original information, the stored blueprint in the DNA (this is the place in the quantum space!), or it can be restored.

However, it is not the water element that is the cause of the imbalance in cancer, but fire! The ancient Chinese rightly spoke of a "sickness of coldness". If the fire of life burns too weakly, if we stop burning for new ideas, the cells lose their sense of maintaining the high degree of coherence (with a lot of effort), and the vicious circle described above begins.

Reproduction is the strongest drive for which a lot of energy is made available (fire element). It is therefore not surprising that regular sex protects against breast and prostate cancer.

With the devices of the Living Systems Information Therapy LSIT, the tumour region is treated directly and additional the functional circuit large intestine / lungs (yellow quadrant), with all information of the blue quadrant (water element). Via the magnetic field / scalar wave application, not only the organs are included locally, but also the meridians.

Every healing process is controlled by the brain, which should be taken into account. The **M**atrix **R**egeneration **T**herapy device **MRT**

503 was specially developed for the biofeedback therapy required for this, with which the matrix is simultaneously deeply cleaned and the environment is renovated. But biofeedback is also easily possible with the Equalizer EQ 103 (Chapter 5.6, page 111).

However, this does not mean that every cancer patient (linear-causal) is treated with the same therapy. Quite the contrary – individuality is taken into account in every respect. 3 + 1 means that the aspect of the water element is used reinforced for therapy, with simultaneous (!) consideration of the other 3 elements.

With regard to the 4 self-esteems acc. *Max Lüscher* (see Fig. 3 p. 39), "personal satisfaction" should be learned and lived, but in interaction with "self-confidence" (red), "self-respect" (green) and "personal freedom" (yellow).

With regard to cell metabolism, HGH (growth hormone, blue) must be activated in the tumour region, but at the same time attention must be paid to the normal function of the adrenal gland (cortisol, yellow), thyroid (thyroxine, red) and anabolic peptides (green) (see Fig. 1 page 16). This takes place automatically as part of the CMR (Cell Milieu Revitalization) treatment, but is also supported by rhythmic movement sequences, carbohydrate restriction and the reduction of permanent psychological stress.

Regarding the neuromodulators, the CMR / Vortex device activates serotonin (blue), but at the same time dopamine, acetylcholine and noradrenaline / adrenaline. This is done automatically using the information stored in analogue form, in accordance with the permanent real-time measurement in the device.

According to this 4-pole principle, to which all body functions are subject, further proven therapy options can be searched and modified accordingly, and used in addition (Chapter 4.7. page 94).

If the selection shows that a means or a method contains only one of the 4 aspects, the other three aspects should be added or, if not possible, this one removed.

Nothing is worse than setting new blockades with one-sided therapies.

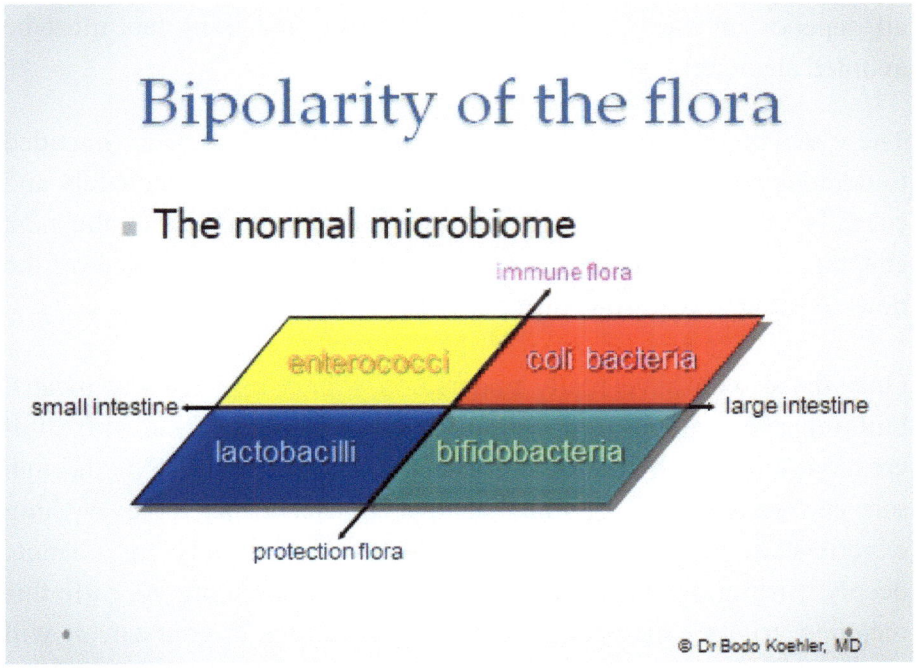

**Fig.4:** Bipolarity of the gut symbionts

Particular attention should also be paid to the structure of the ***intestinal environment*** under appropriate stool controls, as this not only supports the immune system, but also the necessary digestive process (transformation of the cause of loss). Of course, there are also 4-pole interactions here, which should be observed.

The absolutely necessary change in diet also falls into this area, because it has a lasting impact on the inner milieu. Not only should the carbohydrate restriction be mentioned here, but also the guaranteed protein supply, depending on the blood group (A means vegetarian; zero means meat from animals). A lack of proteins with simultaneous carbohydrate fattening significantly hinders healing. It all depends on the right $\Omega$-oils (3 + 1 law), and trans fats must be avoided absolutely (Chapter 1.3.2.).

These therapeutic approaches are detailed later and are only intended to demonstrate the principle that cancer can be treated adequately and causally. The above 6 points indicate the direction. From the next chapter, additional findings will be incorporated that can round off the new understanding of this disease.

Only those who have really understood what LIFE actually means: building a harmonious, loving relationship with oneself and with all of creation, initiating a feeling of connectedness with all BEING through service, readiness for ongoing change, transcendence of everything experienced, never standing still, always being ready for change, deeply trusting the workings of higher laws – and giving your life this meaning, triggers the necessary healing processes in yourself, or will not even get into the situation of a serious illness.

The measure of whether we walk on our path in life or not is the joy we feel in everything we do.

And again: constant change and conversion means constantly create new relationships and trying out possibilities that are offered to us every day anew. Stagnation only occurs through refusal (rejected yellow). Then the essential entanglement with the quantum space (spirit) "loosens", whereby important information is lost.

This also happens through the accumulation of unrelated content (external determination) and substances. Regeneration is then often only partially possible, is carried out incorrectly or leads to uncontrolled growths. Here we come full circle.

## Findings

*'Health is the ability to adapt to changing environmental conditions as quickly as possible'. This theorem by Prof Dr Dr J. Schole assumes a good regulation, namely of the cell metabolism in connection with the acids-base balance. If a chronic illness occurs, the acute, normal defence reaction has resulted in a regulatory blockade.*

*The reasons for the emergence of these interference fields are unprocessed events that were perceived as a threat and created fear. This contaminates the photons that carry life information, which has a negative effect on the tissue structure – up to and including the development of cancer.*

*That is always the case and it gets to the point. What this does not yet answer, however, makes up the main work in a life-supporting practice, namely the WHY.*

*Life is based on constant transformation. Any kind of standstill can be fatal. Life is constantly questioning itself. What is built up may have to be dissolved again in the next moment. 'Life is permanent self-destruction'.*

*The question of the cause can therefore be narrowed down somewhat: Who or what is holding on to the past? Because that's what it's all about. Everything that remains and is not processed is the past.*

*The next aspect is a quantum mechanical one. Mass is only an extremely small part of us. We consist primarily of fields, and these are formed and influenced by our consciousness, because only this is able to release the necessary (structure-forming) energy.*

*Every major event presents a challenge that needs to be addressed, and done immediately. It's about the 'quick' adaptability. Processing cannot take place if the event completely surprised us and caused us to go into shock. Then it ceaselessly circles in our thoughts and imprints itself on our fields. From there it is called up again and again, mostly through similar situations and literally pulls us back into the past like with a fist. Our focus is on it, and we are not free and open to new experiences (yellow in the Luescher cube) to which we can react carefree.*

*This contamination of our organizational fields in the absence of transformation can go so far that cancer develops. The tumour is to be understood as a manifest garbage dump of our constantly circling thoughts, as external information. According to TCM (5 phases of conversion) it can be assigned to specific psychological problems.*

*Healing can only be achieved if these connections lead to a change in consciousness and an active transformation can take place through the affected patient. On this basis, spontaneous healing occurs again and again (one in 10,000). The key to this is to turn away from the disease completely, which should sink it into insignificance, by turning to new tasks and goals. In that way we are destroying the interference with the microbes that have influenced us.*

*The special thing about it is that the cured cancer patients felt (!) completely in agreement with the fact that they will die shortly. This has been the case with all spontaneous healings and is the crucial key. Why is that?*

*'To die' means the dissolution of everything that is and what was. At the same time it is the beginning of a return to our actual origin, namely the spiritual world. This turning to God is called Religio, but it is only achieved by a few during their lifetime. But in the face of death everything material can become totally unimportant, only the spiritual counts.*

*Those who come to this fundamental knowledge early on do not need serious illnesses in order to learn from them, but can lead a fulfilled, carefree life in God-consciousness.*

## 3. Assured new knowledge about development of cancer

Almost 100 years ago, the working group led by Prof Dr *Seyfarth*, MD at the Hospital in Berlin-Buch found *fungi* in all (!) metastases of various types of cancer, sometimes also in the primary tumour.

A little earlier, Prof Dr *F. Boesser*, MD in Hanover postulated a liquid toxic medium that precedes the development of cancer.

Both approaches have in common, that cancer cannot develop, if the cell milieu is not poisoned.

The cancer cell itself arises in an alkaline environment and remains alkaline the whole life. However, through its fermentation metabolism, it gradually creates a strongly acidic environment. This led to the mistake in science that cancer would develop in an acidic environment.

### 3.1 Metabolic dynamics

Dr *Wolfgang Zoech*, MD from Krems (Austria) took the trouble and worked through old publications. The research results are reproduced here in extracts (with kind permission).

*All* cells have 4 different ways of obtaining energy
  ➢ aerobic glycolysis
  ➢ anaerobic glycolysis
  ➢ oxidative phosphorylation
  ➢ Anaerobic chemolithotrophy (energy from organic compounds e.g. $H_2S$). Substances such as glutamine, palmitate, oleate, etc. are metabolized.

Overall, there is an extreme potential for adaptation. Cells are much more flexible to obtain energy than initially expected.

*Epithelial cells stimulate glycolysis in neighbouring fibroblasts.* Lactate / pyruvate push up their mitochondrial phosphorylation. The ATP yield is therefore significantly higher (inverse Warburg effect).

Glycolysis and chemolithotrophy cause high levels of acidity. The inside of the cancer cell, however, requires an *alkaline calibration*. It gets $H_2$ out and bicarbonate into the cell. $H_2CO_3$ is produced by carbonic anhydrase.

**Attention:** *Without carbonic anhydrase*, the cells would die of intoxication! It ensures their survival.

Germ cells migrate through the embryo from the end of the 3rd week. Only about 30% reach the germination line, the "rest" is distributed. Later, these are the *adult stem cells* on the basement membranes. They divide 10-15 times and differentiate into organ cells.

## Caution: Differentiated cells are unable to divide!

The telomere length at birth is approximately 10,000 base pairs. Each division shortens them. At 4000 the so-called *Hayflick limit* is reached. The limit is shown by the external aging of around 40 years. Gentle immune stimulation counteracts this (e.g. sun).

The risk of cancer increases with decreasing telomere length. If a cell reaches its limit during division, it stops. It remains as a *not completely differentiated cell*. If it affects many cells, the result is inferior tissue, e.g. leucoplakia, broad-based polyps, cysts or anaplasias.

As a result, it happens earlier and earlier. *Embryonic tissue* is created.

The decrease in the degree of differentiation is called *re-feotalization*. This can go as far as the *embryonic trophoblast cell*. This corresponds to a tumour stem cell. There is a changed set of chromosomes.

**Attention:** Chemotherapy promotes and accelerates this process!

At the Hayflick limit, the stem cell becomes apoptotic (optimum), or it becomes age rigid, i.e. passive without division (coldness > ATP↓). In this *replicative senescence* it produces inflammatory substances. The resulting inflammation promotes cancer.

## Cancer can arise from adult re-foetalized stem cells.

*The development of a cancerous tumour can be understood as a consequence of a disturbed, incomplete differentiation!*
But cell *regeneration* also starts in this state. Each renewal corresponds to a partial embryogenesis. The cell *milieu* alone makes the difference!

Coldness and heavy metal deposits are ideal conditions for fungal growth. Fungi were found in tumours and metastases to 99%. They block the necessary organ information from the surrounding cell milieu. This triggers survival reflexes in the *isolated* senescent cell.
A nutrient germ (trophoblast) is formed. The senescent cell mutates into cancer stem cell.

**3.2. Fungi** (origin Wikipedia)
"Fungi cannot photosynthesize. They feed by ingesting organic substances. They absorb these in dissolved form from the environment. Fungi are more closely related to animals than to plants. There are protozoa with many nuclei (syncytium).

Fungi are the oldest living creation in the world. They spread extremely quickly. The fungi hyphae (in the soil) are *immortal*. Fungi can take different forms in humans. Some types contain cures for cancer (Lentinan, Crestin).

Fungi have an anaerobic metabolism and give off $CO_2$. The mycelium (network) can become hard permanent forms. Their way of life is *parasitic, corrosive, or symbiotic.*

Not every parasite kills its host. Weak parasites only attack previously damaged hosts. Examples are the Maitake, which is coveted as medicinal fungus, and the Reishi. The 'Hedgehog prickly beard' is rarer, but important in medicine.

The 'Chaga' or 'Crooked Schillerporling' has a strong healing power, also the 'Rattlesponge'. "

Further to the remarks by *W. Zoech:*

The cancer stem cell increases its glycolytic program and produces large amounts of lactic acid (which helps the fungi). The carbonic anhydrase is ramped up to the maximum: $CO_2 + H2O \rightarrow H_2CO_3$.

The telomeres shorten to a minimum. Due to the threat of cell death, a big amount of telomerase is released.

## There is much to suggest that cancerous tumours are the enslavement of senescent adult stem cells by fungi!

Cancer stem cells are emigrated primordial germ cells that suddenly emulate their sister cells in the gonads. A carcinoma is a "parthenogenetic" trophoblast (virgin procreation).

According to *F. Boesser*, every infection – but also cancer – needs a "fire accelerator". *Fungi and special poisons* are, according to him, the unknown missing link. Toxic *alkaloids* transform the *environment* hostile to life. The damaged cells want to break out through growth. The *loss of control of the brain* due to the lack of afferent nerve fibres is essential for understanding!

Local *lymph congestion and blood stasis* (also due to cardiac insufficiency) have a supporting effect. The para-inflammatory oedema intensifies this effect. The toxic fungal serum is constantly changing (also according to Prof Dr *Enderlein*). Bacteria and viruses are to be understood as intermediate stages. Tubercle bacteria can, for example, turn into 'Radiation Fungi' (Actinomycosis). *Tuberculosis can trigger leukaemia!*

### 3.2.1. Fungi poisons (origin Wikipedia)

Mycotoxins include

> ➢ Aflatoxins
> ➢ Alternaria toxins
>> ▪ Alternariol (AOH)
>> ▪ Alternariol monomethyl ether (AME)
>> ▪ Altenuen and tenuazonic acid
> ➢ Fusarium toxins
>> ▪ Trichothecenes
> ➢ Deoxynivalenol (DON)
> ➢ Nivalenol
> ➢ T-2 toxin
>> ▪ Zearalenone
>> ▪ Fumonisins
> ➢ Ochratoxins (Aspergillus, Penicillium)
> ➢ Ergot alkaloids (ergot alkaloids)

**3.2.1.1. Alkaloids** (origin Wikipedia)
> ➢ Ergot alkaloids: e.g. secale cornutum, ergotamine, ergometrine
> ➢ Curare alkaloids: e.g. toxiferin, tubocurarine, alcuronium
> ➢ Opiates: e.g. morphine, codeine, thebaine, papaverine, noscapine, cryptopine
> ➢ Vinca alkaloids: e.g. vincristine, vinblastine
> ➢ Lobelia alkaloids: e.g. lobeline, lelobanidine, lobelanidine
> ➢ Strychnos alkaloids: e.g. akuammicin, brucine, strychnine
> ➢ Catharanthus alkaloids: e.g. catharanthine, vindoline
> ➢ Amaryllidaceae alkaloids: e.g. lycorine, galantamine
> ➢ Dendrobates alkaloids: e.g. histrionicotoxin, pumiliotoxin
> ➢ Lupine alkaloids: e.g. lupinine, lupanine, sparteine
> ➢ China alkaloids: e.g. quinine, quinidine
> ➢ Coca alkaloids: e.g. cocaine, ecgonine, hygrine

Cholesterol

Example for alkaloid

Epigallocatechin can be used as an antidote (green tea extract), also tannin

It is noticeable that many of the alkaloids are *steroids* and can resemble cholesterol. This makes them cavity resonators for photons (storage) and can develop disruptive hormonal effects. Others can have a positive effect, e.g. quinine.

### 3.2.1.2. Effects (origin Wikipedia)

*Mycotoxins* can have toxic effects on humans and animals even in low concentrations.

- ➤ In particular, mycotoxins
    - o have a carcinogenic effect
    - o damage the central nervous system (neurotoxic)
    - o damage the immune system (immunosuppressive)
    - o damage the genetic material (mutagenic)
    - o damage the fruit of the womb (teratogenic effect)
    - o cause organ damage (e.g. liver or kidney) (have a hepatotoxic or nephrotoxic effect)
- ➤ Cause skin and mucous membrane damage (from skin irritation to necrosis) on contact,
- ➤ Inhibit or initiate enzymatic metabolic processes
- ➤ Trigger allergic reactions,
- ➤ Cause fertility disorders through *hormonal effects*.

### 3.3. Coccidia (origin Wikipedia)

"In a host cell, usually in the gastrointestinal tract, blood, liver or kidney, they carry out asexual reproduction in the form of a schizogony / merogony (splitting) through multiple nuclear divisions and thereby destroy the cell.

Each of the so-called merozoites (up to 100 from a parent cell) then infects a new cell and the process is repeated.

The form of division depends on the parasite: ***Toxoplasma gondii*** divides in a form called endodyogeny, while Eimeria has a schizogony / merogony division pattern.

In ***Sarcocystis*** the pattern of division is called endopolygonia." (According to Prof *Adamkiewicz*, they are the cause of Colon-Ca.)

## Microbes are able to change our personality and influence our actions!

Wikipedia: "The number of asexual reproductions is specific for each coccidia species. Following the asexual phase of reproduction (schizogony), sex cells (gametogony) form, namely large plasma-rich macrogametes and small flagellated microgametes, and sexual reproduction takes place.

The fertilized female cell (zygote) surrounds itself with a shell (encystation) and becomes an oocyst. It is excreted with the host's faeces.

In the outside world there is reduction division (meiosis), in which mononuclear division products (sporoblasts) form and surround themselves with shells, the so-called spores (sporogony).

The infectious sporozoites form in the spores with a further division (mitosis).

In ***Sarcocystis***, the sporulation already takes place in the host, the oocyst envelope breaks open before leaving the intestine and sporocysts are excreted" (end of quote).

## 3.4. Step by step program

Up to this point it has become clear that fungi are an essential cofactor in the development and maintenance of cancer. But it is not yet clear where these come from and what causes them to spread inside the body.

We're talking about the intestines first. Fungi look for niches on our mucous membranes. These are places with a reduced mucus layer and without surface colonization of our protective flora. These voids can be the result of antibiotic treatments or toxic damage.

However, this is not enough to open the door to the inside for the fungi. Special circumstances are necessary: Due to a lack of gastric acid (mostly blood group A, or caused by acid blockers), the pH value shifts upwards. Under these conditions our normal flora cannot live and is reduced. The empty spaces are occupied by putrefactive bacteria (clostridia, enter bacteria, etc.). These metabolize all types of protein. This creates ammonia, which further intensifies the alkalosis.

Ammonia is extremely toxic, especially to the liver and brain.

80% of the immune system is located in the small intestine and is in close cooperation with the healthy intestinal bacteria (Fig. 4 page 58). If these are missing or reduced, this naturally has an effect on the defence performance. This can promote bacterial infections. This is the chance for fungi!

In the course of such an inflammation, the invading bacteria smuggle the fungi with them into the depths. The immune system can then largely eliminate the bacteria, but not the fungi. It is rarely able to do this.

The fungal nests form mainly in hard-to-reach areas with reduced blood flow and poor lymphatic drainage. Old areas of inflammation, which are usually acidic, are particularly suitable for this.

These could not heal because in most cases (heavy) metal deposits are located there, which stress the matrix and permanently disrupt its function as a dielectric.

But this is by no means a mechanical process. This scenario has a long history! Since our brain monitors all areas of the body, these depots would have been thwarted from the start, because dealing with parasites has been diligently practiced for thousands of years.

There is only one suitable explanation for this, and that is loss of control by the brain through damage to afferent fibres!

A few situations in life are responsible for this: infections with *neurotoxic viruses*, e.g. Epstein-Barr, varicella zoster, herpes simplex, especially HHV VI, but also *vaccine damage* caused by toxic pathogens.

But not only that: Thimerosal (mercury) in the vaccinations itself has a neurotoxic effect. Frequently vaccinated people are therefore particularly at risk. Mercury also blocks the lymphatic system.

Unfortunately, not enough attention is paid to the de-myelination of nerve fibres by *mobile communications!*

These pre-damaged areas only give weak or *no feedback* at all to the brain, which is a prerequisite for autonomous processes, i.e. fungal nests, inflammation centres, and even cancer.

But not only the lack of a control function by the brain, but also the collapse of the 'maser hologram' enables the pathological transformation of the tissue (Chapter 4.5.1. page 91).

The loss of nerve fibres has been proven several times – also by *Thomas Tallberg* in Finland – if only one was looking for it!

One point is still missing and that is the operating temperature. If it falls below 36.5° C (97.7° F) at these points, the mitochondria switch off and no longer produce ATP. These are ideal conditions for microbes (colds!) to spread, which we always carry around on our mucous membranes anyway. Unfortunately, this is often mistaken for an infection. However, it is nothing more than a constellation that results from the interaction of several factors under certain conditions (see Fig. 5).

With these new points of view, we need to set a much longer period for cancer development, starting in childhood.
Anyone who was vaccinated before they were one year old and then received *a lot of vaccinations* later on is predisposed to developing cancer later on. This has nothing to do with a vaccination opposition, but is simply a fact.

This first stage is usually followed by many years without any problems. Then can an infection (better "contamination") with the widespread neurotoxic viruses occur, which – depending on the location – damage the local nerve network and thus prepare the ground for the second stage – the *loss of control through the brain*. In a state of full health, the current state is constantly checked in every area of the body and kept in balance through compensatory measures.

All regeneration processes are coordinated via the autonomic nervous system, but this requires precise feedback.
A chronic focus of inflammation is favored by metal deposits in the tissue, because this disrupts the semiconductor function of the matrix

and thus the flow of electrons. But its emergence already indicates a loss of control.

When it comes to the settlement of fungi nests, the proof is provided. Fungi are the worst form of hostile takeover. This can be observed very beautifully in nature on dying trees. The body would defend itself against this with all its might – if he knew about it!

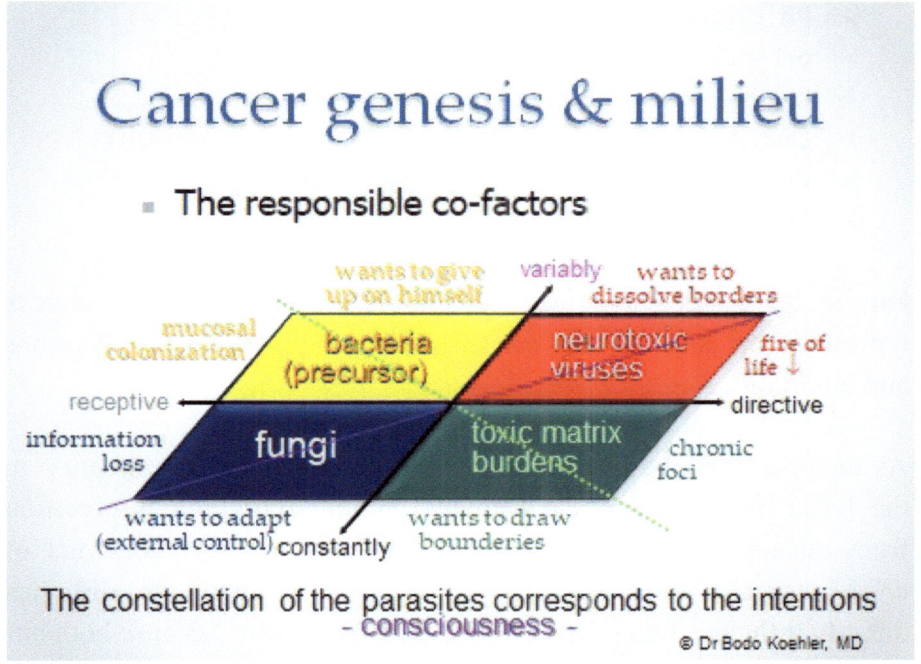

**Fig.5:** The responsible co-factors seen holistically

Fungi take every chance to multiply. And now a race against the cells begins. The development of the cancer tumor is therefore an attempt to break out of isolation by the fungi and the associated loss of information. This is explained in detail in the various chapters.

71

### 3.4.1. Fungi-friendly terrain
- ➤ Moist and warm
- ➤ Weakened immune system
- ➤ Hormonal changes!
- ➤ Depots of heavy metals or aluminium
- ➤ Toxic burdens by environmental toxins
- ➤ Foci of inflammation, with or without microbes
- ➤ Lymph congestion
- ➤ Poor blood supply, lack of oxygen
- ➤ pH shift
- ➤ Lack of light (loss of photons due to de-coherence)
- ➤ Degenerative diseases (catabolic metabolic derailment)
- ➤ Psychological problems > self-abandonment
- ➤ Loss of authenticity

Not to be neglected is the psychological situation, which always represents the level of our *consciousness*, with its goals, intentions and emotions.

As interesting as the observation of the microbes and the situation in the tissue may be, nothing happens without retrieving information from quantum space (top-down). All of creation is a construct of consciousness. We create reality through our intentions and thus directly influence other forms of life. This is possible because both our DNA and their DNA are in the quantum state and are therefore able to exchange information. However, this can also go in the wrong direction, as microbes influence our psyche (e.g. toxoplasmosis).

According to these explanations, it is not surprising if the tissue cells in such an area no longer behave normally and start to proliferate.

Because these milieu changes can isolate cell aggregates. They lose contact and the indispensable opportunity to exchange information.

### 3.4.2. Loss of communication
➢ Stem cells constantly communicate with the tissue
➢ If there is no answer from there, it is a division signal
➢ The condition for new, **unchecked** growth is **isolation**
➢ This then leads to a loss of control in the brain (no feedback)
➢ Congestion of electrons lead to a very alkaline tissue
➢ The mitochondria need a lot of protons (acid)
➢ ATP synthesis cannot start > cell potential drops
➢ Division is only possible to a limited extent

This leads to small, non-functional cells → catabolic derailment.

### 3.4.3. Loss of relationship
➢ The condition for new, **unchecked** growth is **isolation**
➢ Loss of relationship means sudden loss of information
➢ Loss of information leads to (unstructured) increase in mass
➢ The information gaps are filled by parasites
➢ This can lead to cell enslavement
➢ The cell **milieu** alone decides what the future will look like
➢ An **external** change in the environment creates a new context
➢ As a result, awareness sets new priorities
➢ Isolation is replaced by **new relationships**
➢ New goals and tasks give birth to courage to live

### 3.4.4. Disturbance field and its meaning
➢ No illness without an interference field!
➢ Herd indicate a disturbance of the structural information,
➢ No interference field without stressful emotions! (Timeline)

> ➤ Fear → entry KIDNEY → brain → holographic network
> ➤ ***De-myelination of nerve fibres by mobile communications!***
> ➤ Loss of control by the brain
> ➤ Metal deposits → dielectric↓ > parasites↑

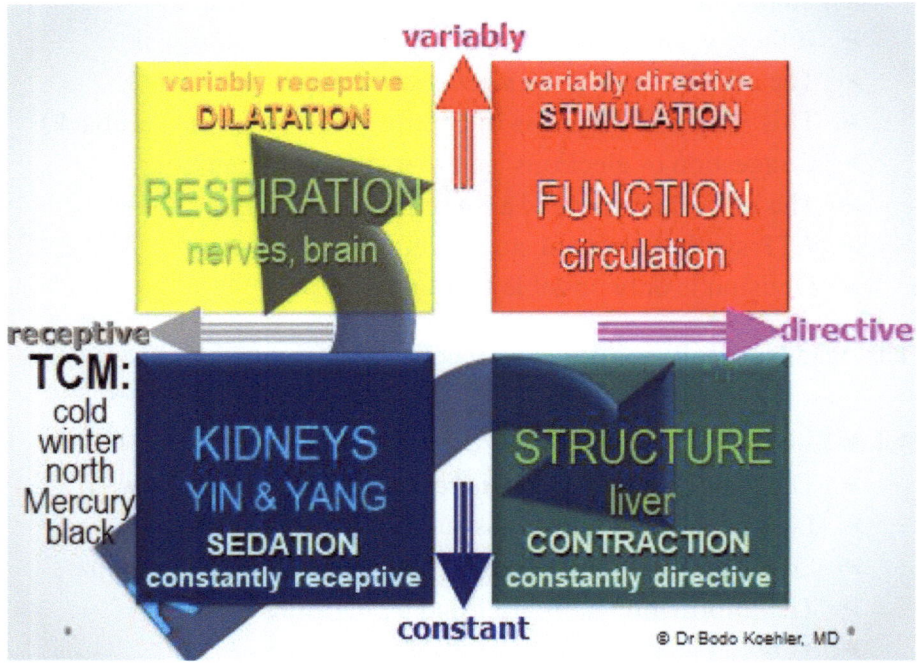

**Fig.6:** The kidneys as a central distributor of information

### 3.4.5. Loss of binding

> ➤ Cancer means disturbed internal ***breathing***
> ➤ Cancer means a destroyed tissue ***structure***
> ➤ Cancer is a lack of control by the ***brain***
> ➤ Cancer is a kidney problem!
> ➤ Kidney contains origin information
> ➤ Kidney means basic trust

> The kidney is the seat of life energy
> *Kidney secures existence through binding!*
> Binding means increased coherence
> Binding means *LOVE*

Every disturbance field shows a kidney disorder – parts of the soul are not developed. *Kidney information* serves to *maintain the structure* as a prerequisite for *function*. They thus form the interface to the separation axis (liver).

As part of the *neural functional model* (Chap. 4.5.1.), the kidneys also control the yellow and green quadrants in the Luescher cube and, via the integration axis, the red one (energy release =).

The kidneys also form the resting point in the organism in order to reach the quantum mechanical ground state. This is a prerequisite for every healing process. Existential fear, as the main burden in the sense of TCM, prevents this. Creating trust is therefore one of the main tasks of the doctor.

## 3.5. Form and function

> No function without form
> Form is created by *flowing in opposite directions*
> A pulsating magnetic field is created arterially
> This produces a rhythmic e-field venous
> Ionized molecules are transported electrically
> Cancer has no venous drainage!
> The tissue produces a *landfill*
> The magnetic field predominates, the electrical field is weak
> The discrepancy between a strong m-field (e-smog!) and too few charge carriers promotes cancer growth → loss of structure
> The reason is *insufficient ionization energy*

> The rhythmic circulation of the blood is shifted in favour of flowing in

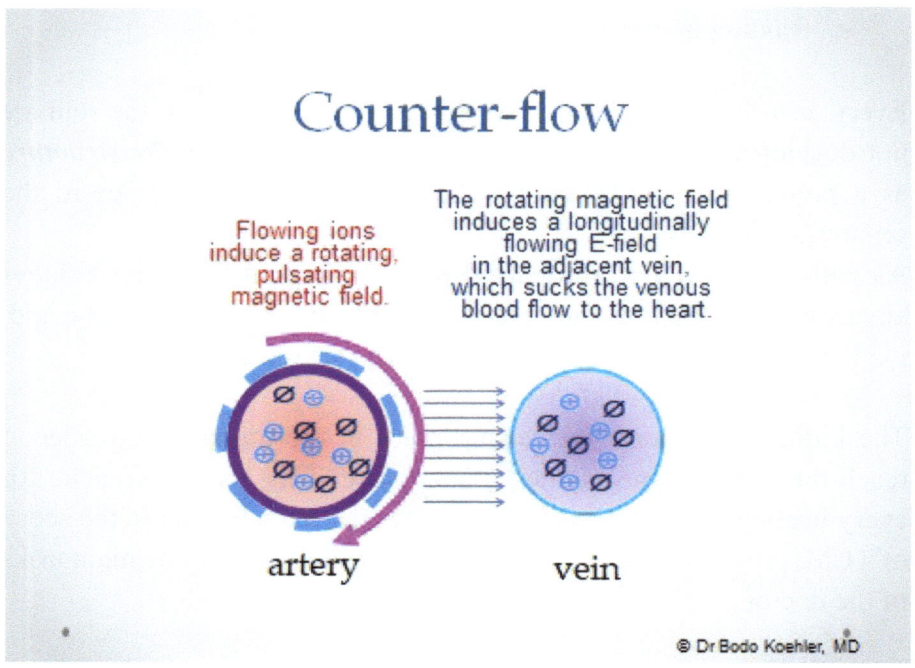

**Fig. 7:** Loss of charge creates cancer-promoting stasis

Cancer doesn't grow, but spreads as healthy cells are recruited and cancer stem cells immigrate. Even cells of the immune system (macrophages in M2 mode) are reprogrammed into cancer cells. This is favored by heat and energy loss.

The sun plays a major role here, since we are light beings and without sufficient photons, no information transmission is possible.

US pathologist Prof Dr Frank Apperly, MD 1941: "The more sun, the less cancer".

## 3.6. Mitochondria

*Opening* through:
- ➢ NO, $CO_2$, acetyl-l-carnitine
- ➢ 420 nm λ (UV light)

*Closure* by:
- ➢ **Calcium**, CO, cooling below 36.5° C (97.7° F)
- ➢ 450 nm λ (violet light)

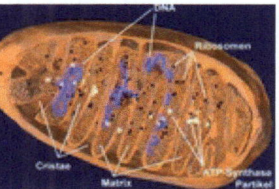

# Power station

## Mitochondria

- number 2500 – 3500/cell in the youth
- personal genome (from mother), can mutate more easily existing damage was transferred from the mother
- reasons: Lack of Mg!, Zn, Cu, „Vitamin" D, C, E, $B_{3, 6, 9, 12}$ heavy metals, Fe↑ pestizids, bact., viruses, fungus micro wave radiation, handy, antennas, cordless
- ATP level is controlled in the carotides
- increase due to physical work and light exposure!
- NF-kappaB (inflammat.) induces Survivin > stops apoptosis
- electron leak creates radicals (carbohydrates↓!!!)

© Dr Bodo Koehler, MD

**Fig.8:** Overview of relevant factors of the mitochondria

**There are 2 genomes in the cell**
- ➢ The archaic cell genome A (DNA) is the older one
- ➢ The mitochondria genome B (circular) is younger

> ➢ Genome B dominates cell genome A (DNA)
> ➢ With cancer cells it is the opposite:
> ➢ DNA controls (predominantly) energy production in cytoplasm

**Changes caused by this:**
> ➢ Decrease in the thiol pool (glutathione, cysteine)
> ➢ Shift in the redox equilibrium → oxidation
> ➢ Consequence: mitochondrial insufficiency and loss of dominance of the B genome
> ➢ This is due to a lack of protons and thyroxine

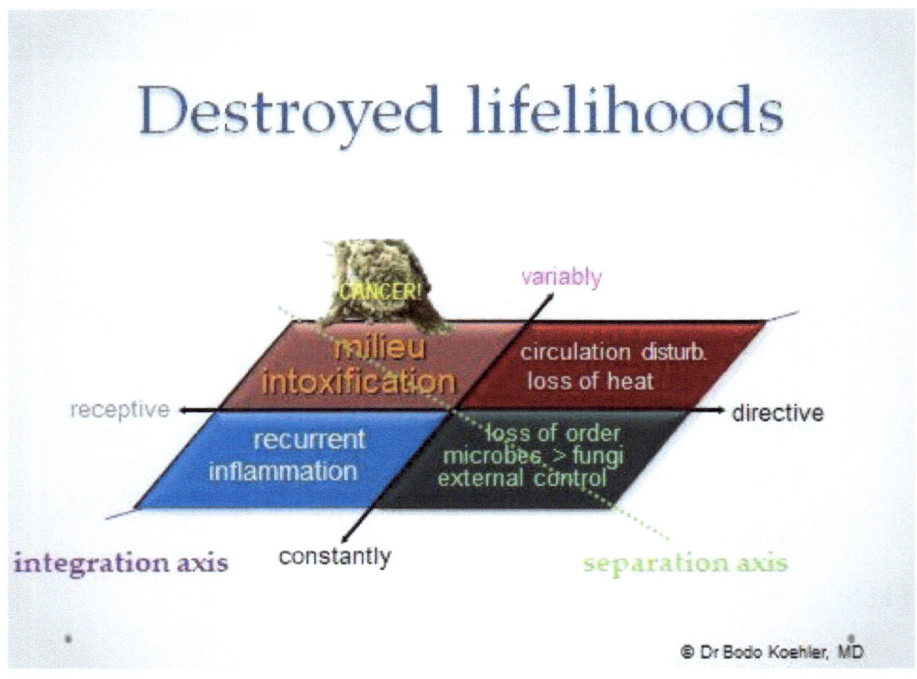

**Fig.9:** Tissue changes as a prerequisite for cancer genesis

## 3.7. Psychological characteristics

➢ Illness: blood poisoning by imbalance – cancer too!
➢ Discrepancy between perception & understanding → bipolar disorder
➢ This loss of authenticity is felt with fear
➢ The sense of facts is no longer revealed (no bottom-up)
➢ Critical questioning turns into blind faith
➢ Luescher diagnostics: isolation in the yellow quadrant (= environment)
➢ ++ 4: "excessive hope and expectation for the future"
➢ - - 4: "my INABILITY to allow changes and to adjust to new things" (original text by *M. Luescher*)
➢ The separation axis has derailed due to paradoxical behaviour in the ***green quadrant*** (see Fig. 1 and 3)
➢ The (reciprocal) integration axis cannot compensate
➢ Blue is not in balance with red
➢ ***Transformation of external signals is disturbed***
➢ Red is overtaxed > blue needs support (water)
➢ Loss of information (blue) means loss of structure → increase in mass
➢ In the timeless quantum state (spirit) there is high potentiality
➢ Room information and cell information interact
➢ ***Everything*** is possible; limitation by lack of imagination and fear (- - 4, yellow quadrant)
➢ The gene sequence is read in a meaningful manner

## 3.8. Co-factors in the development

➢ Suppressed ***needs of the soul*** (Prof *Grossarth-Maticek*)
➢ Permanent focus on the disease (→ insignificance!)
➢ ***Isolation*** (real or felt)
➢ Constant conflict, depressive loss syndrome, diabolical fear

➤ Unprocessed shock → the "path" was left beforehand
➤ Lack of meaning in life / life task
➤ Escape from life (yellow); Loss of authenticity (green) Fig.1+3
➤ Epiphyseal calcification (Gl. pinealis) → contact interruption
➤ Wrong nutrition (carbohydrate fattening) → *fungi!* Zinc↓ (vegetarian)
➤ *Hormones* (wrong breakdown pathways in the liver), trans fats
➤ Allopathics, harmful food supplements: "vitamin" D, calcium, alkaline powder aggravates
➤ Fatty liver (NAFLD) toxins → *lack of flowing electricity in connective tissue*; geopathy, *electro smog*
➤ Gastric acid deficiency → B12 deficiency > anaemia
➤ *Parasite infestation (fungi, coccidia, bacteria, viruses)*
➤ Iodine deficiency (almost all organs) → thyroxine deficiency
➤ Lack of heat (ionization energy), *hypothyroidism*
➤ *Sun deficiency* (Prof *Apperly*: Sun deficiency disease!)
➤ Electron maldistribution (too little fresh organic food)
➤ Magnesium and potassium deficiency, calcium excess

Some hints of treatment options have already suggested. This is discussed and continued in Chapter 4.7. from page 94.

But it should already become clear that a resounding success can only be achieved with a sophisticated, individualized concept that takes all facets into account.

This includes the *elimination of local stasis* that promote fungal growth (lowering blood pressure is counterproductive here), namely with increasing the heart rate (high dose of iodine) by stimulating the thyroid gland (with cardiac support: digitalis, strophanthin), increasing the ionization energy through the application of heat, but also the active stimulation of *counter-flow* through local, pulse-controlled application of direct current (by LYMPHO*DYN*®).

Of course, the psychological aspect and the active raising of body heat are still missing. This is also discussed in a later chapter. The only aim here is to first awaken a feeling that this is a completely new view and therefore a completely different therapeutic approach that fully takes into account the four-pole, mutual influence – the bipolar interaction – that is evident in all areas of life. It can be seen at the Luescher cube and is very easy to understand. Bacteria and viruses are also in a polar relationship and influence each other, just like fungi and heavy metals perpendicular to this (Fig. 5 on page 71). Mercury, for example, is often found in candida nests.

Despite all effective measures, the patient should be actively involved in the therapy and consistently reorganize his life.

Healing works spontaneously when the unshakable belief in God's healing love has become established knowledge and results in the conviction of a *safe healing*.

Inner peace – wanting nothing, asking for nothing, personal satisfaction – is a prerequisite for every healing process. In order to achieve this, the following measures are helpful:

### 3.9. Quantum mechanical ground state QMG
- Conflict resolution!
- Stress reduction on all levels, focus cleansing, detoxification
- Flat renovation: geopathy, e-smog, wooden beds, foam mattresses…
- Accepting the situation, let it happen, don't fight!
- Embody the meaning of existence as a total system
- Occupy & defend the space, experience yourself as a whole
- Coherence therapy with MRT 503 or ZMR 703

➤ Meditation, Pray
➤ Yoga
➤ Classical music
➤ Bathing in warm salt water (primordial sea)
➤ Visiting places of power
➤ Forest walks

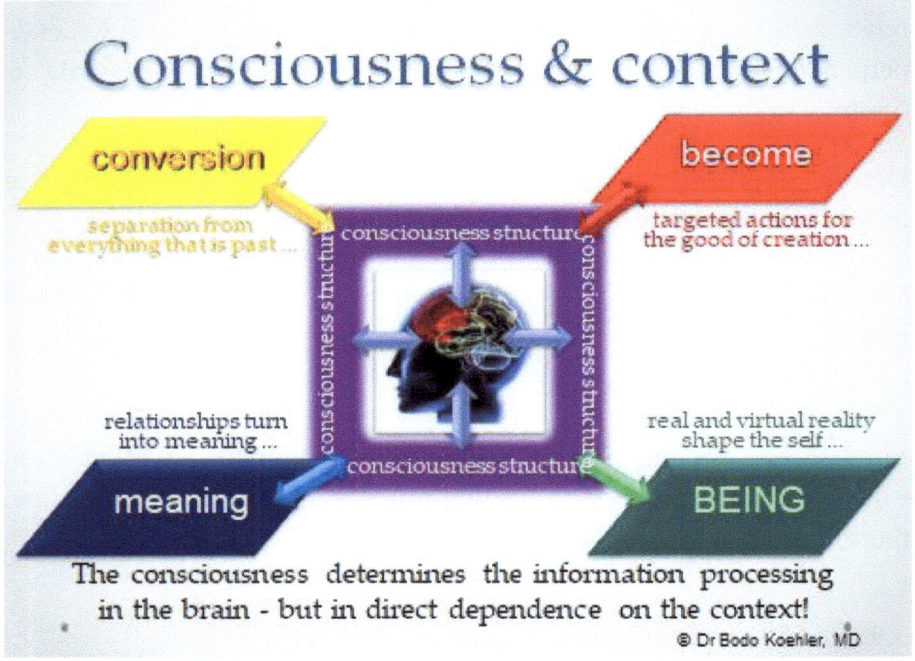

**Fig.10:** Consciousness serves the whole from a higher sense

### 3.9.1. Control function of the brain
➤ Transverse flooding with short wave (acc. to Dr *Schliephake*)
➤ Polarity reversal of the direct current system (NEC 708)
➤ Local correction of cell metabolism (according to Prof *Schole*)
➤ Transfer of the tumour information with Equalizer EQ 103 or MRT 503 to the corresponding brain region (feedback!)

### 3.9.2. Realignment
> ➢ Context!
> ➢ Redesign of the room, change of place, change of residence ...
> ➢ Enthusiasm for new goals, tasks for life (yellow)
> ➢ No worries anymore, living to the limit (red)
> ➢ Spin-flip: living in unconditional love in God (blue)
> ➢ ***Developing a servant awareness for God's Kingdom***

**Findings**

*A cardinal error in cancer research is the focussing on the tumour. However, it can only arise if the cell environment is poisoned.*

*Inadequate detoxification (measures) burden(s) the matrix. Wrong nutrition, environmental toxins and **electro smog** are the main evils.*

*Local lymph congestion, microcirculation disturbance, oxygen deficiency, $CO_2$ enrichment, light and electron deficiency are ideal conditions for fungal growth; coldness, chronic foci and heavy metal deposits have an intensifying effect. Bacteria and viruses play the role of co-factors. They can trigger the spread of fungi.*

*But nothing of the kind would be possible if the brain had not lost its control function. Local, toxic nerve degeneration is responsible for this. Vaccination damage and subsequent virus infections can cause this, but so can cell phones.*

*Fungi toxins paralyze the nervous system and damage the immune system, liver and kidneys. Fungi isolate cell clusters, thus preventing communication. The cells try to restart through growth. The cancer tumour can therefore be understood as a second embryo.*

*Fungi and other parasites are only indicators of the poisoned environment and loss of control. Antimycotics or the like are therefore counterproductive. Only the thorough renovation of the cell milieu can stand up to this cutthroat competition.*

*Fixation on the tumour (every examination!) prevents transformation. The "blood poisoning through imbalance" demands regulation on all levels. In addition to therapeutic measures, transcendence is necessary. Nothing happens without a higher meaning. Every illness is the visible expression that this patient has not followed his destiny and has left the path.*

*Healing is always possible with a targeted selection from the above measures! However, this presupposes the willingness for changes and the realignment of life on the part of the patient – which is often not wanted!*

*Already at this point it becomes clear that diseases do not only take place on a material level. There are always several facets that intertwine like compartments. In this way, the development of cancer can also be understood as a complex, dynamic process. This has the advantage that we do not have to treat all levels, but only those to which we have the best access. Nevertheless, it always has an effect on the overall process.*

*Patients to whom we have a "good connection" will be easier to reach on the mental level than purely materialistically oriented sick people who respond better to "technical" methods such as physical therapy or infusions.*

# 4. Attempt to structure

Under the aspect that cancer is to be seen as a logical consequence of an insufficient ability to detoxify, with the result of a toxic matrix load, resulting in a loss of control through the brain, and then it is unmistakably clear where a successful therapy has to start. But there are many options. That's why I'm trying with a structure.

## The 4 factors that cause cancer
  - ➤ *No* cancer without loss of control through the brain
    - Nerve degeneration by toxins, vaccinations, viruses, cell phones
  - ➤ *No* cancer without sufficient ionization energy > electr.charge↓
    - Lack of heat > lack of charge carriers > lymph congestion, ATP↓
  - ➤ *No* cancer without matrix poisoning and foci of inflammation
    - All deposits destroy the dielectric
  - ➤ *No* cancer without parasite infestation > loss of information
    - Fungi, among other things, isolate the trophoblasts

## 4.1. Body heat

37° C (98.6° F) body temperature is the basis for all metabolic processes. No more ATP is formed as soon as the temperature drops below 36.5° C (97.7° F).

In this context, the ionization energy comes into focus because the molecules can only be processed in the ionized state. During the synthesis, the individual building blocks are ordered and brought together via electrical field lines.

The ability to produce enough heat when needed was lost in most cancer patients long before the onset of the disease. When asked when they last had a fever, they often have to think for a long time.
Incidentally, cancer is considered a cold sickness in TCM.

The thyroid is responsible for body heat. She comes to the fore in all considerations. The population not only has a serious deficiency in magnesium, but also in iodine. This is due to the fact that not only the thyroid but almost all organ cells have iodine receptors. The liver cells even have two. The intake through food is therefore not sufficient, since the total requirement is in the range of milligrams (instead of micrograms). In addition, few people eat sea fish every day. Because of the associated heavy metal pollution, this is not recommended either.

The thyroid function can be measured quite well by the temperature sensation. Those who freeze easily have a problem. With the laboratory values, it should be ensured that the standard value for TSH, contrary to the usual information, is between 0.8 and 1.2, no more and no less.

Selenium, zinc and progesterone should also be determined, as deficiencies also affect thyroxine production.

Conversely, it becomes understandable why heat applications, e.g. red light, but especially hyperthermia, have such good effects. In the sauna, there is an additional effect – hormesis through the strong cooling stimulus.

## 4.2. Microcirculation and lymph

Not only the detoxification performance depends on the normal body temperature, but also the microcirculation. If the blood pressure is too low or the heart is weak, local blood stasis occurs, which is additionnally promoted by cold (vascular constriction), but also by local acid (focus). This is exacerbated by a lack of fluids and a lack of exercise.

Because the oxygen supply also depends on the blood circulation, pH shifts are to be expected in these areas. These changes in the milieu weaken the immune system and prepare the ground for parasites, especially fungi.

There must therefore be a primary interest in getting the lymph and microcirculation going again. As shown in Fig. 7 page 76, the charge carriers play the decisive role here. Therefore, the previous point gains additional importance, because without ionization energy, these are not sufficiently available.

Another necessity is the arterially induced electric field for the venous return transport, which can only develop inadequately with poor circulation. External stimulation with pulsed direct current can be helpful here (e.g. LYMPHO*DYN*®).

### 4.3. The matrix as a dielectric
When studying medicine, physics is only part of the training up to the first big exam, which is a huge mistake. Many body functions are based on physical processes and can only be understood and interpreted with the appropriate knowledge.

The human being is an electrical system that is kept under tension by differences in charge. Only with death do all charges collapse. In inflammatory processes, this happens much earlier locally, which explains the transition to degeneration.

The matrix functions as a semiconductor due to its silica content. It not only allows electrons to flow in a certain direction, but also acts as an electron store (dielectric). Deposits can destroy this property, especially metals. The connective tissue matrix can then no longer fulfil its task as a basic regulatory system.

In this context, particular attention should be paid to denatured fats (acc. to Johanna Budwig) as well as heavy metals and, of course, foci of inflammation (see Chapter 3.4.4. page 73).

Thorough cleaning and rehabilitation of the matrix is therefore essential for every healing process (see Chapter 4.7.1. page 96).

### 4.4. Parasites

The awareness of parasites was only brought back to the public through *Hulda Clark*. In the past, scabies, fleas, lice, worms and others were part of life – when there was a lack of hygiene. Fungi were less present because they can only be seen under a microscope.

Nevertheless, they have always played a major role. The best-known representatives include candida albicans and the much more dangerous aspergillus flavus (mold) – compare Chapter 3.2. page 62.

The Swiss fungi researcher *Bruno Haefeli* had compiled extensive material for decades and made videos about the spread in the organism, the frightening thing being the speed and its versatility. They can adapt to any milieu and survive as spores for millennia (see pharaohs tombs).

Unfortunately, we have to give up the illusion that effective fungal therapy is possible. We do not hit them with the known antimycotics, but only induce a different, much more resistant form of life.

Paroli can only be offered through a healthy cell milieu that offers our immune system the best conditions to keep the tissue free from microbes. But with increasing age, this succeeds less and less. We must therefore finally accept that fungi do not represent an infection in our body, but that it is a permanent state – a forced symbiosis – which is becoming more and more normal because fungi use every niche that is released and where they can spread out.

Some fungi are quite useful. However, all of the endogenous forms known to date are harmful, and in some cases extreme. They produce toxins (see 3.2.1. and 3.2.1.1), which are strong cell poisons. At the same time, they lead to an isolation of the cells, which are thereby cut off from the exchange of information with the neighbouring cells.

**Coccidia** have similar negative effects, but are only localized in the colon, which is why Prof *Albert Adamkiewicz* (University of Vienna) considered them to be a co-factor in colon cancer, especially the form of sarcocystis.

### 4.4.1. Isolation
This term plays a key role in the development of cancer. As *W. Zoech* already pointed out, we have to start from an embryonic trophoblast that gives rise to the tumour, just as stem cells grow into tissue cells. However, with the difference that immigrated stem cells can be supplied with the necessary information for differentiation by the neighbouring cells, but the trophoblast isolated by fungi cannot.

The information transfer takes place with so-called Energy & Information Exchange Complexes EIEC. This is a gas of $\pi$-electrons, which contain information-carrying solar photons, or which have arisen from them under certain, very sensitive resonance conditions (see Fig.2 page 23). Fungi (and other parasites) can significantly disrupt these information fields because they oscillate very coherently.

At this point it must be clearly emphasized that all bodily functions represent aspects of consciousness that are not possible without a medium mediating between matter and spirit. In quantum mechanics one starts from a quantum state, which is essential for the functioning of our soul.

Our soul drives us by *needs* in order to live to the fullest and to gain experience. This includes many changing relationships at all levels and intensive communication. Every refusal out of fear of life, every self-withdrawal up to isolation, is absolutely harmful to health. It can also be sudden events through loss. Such uprooting can trigger cancer. It is not uncommon, that these patients create the wish to die.

Fear reduction, dealing with trauma, shock resolution and the generation of new trust are central components of every therapy.

### 4.5. Neural control loop

All states and all actions in the organism are reported to the brain via afferent fibres. Amazingly, fewer or no connections to the spinal cord were found in patients with breast cancer! This information deficit must automatically lead to incorrect control. Increased growth signals are to be expected because the area in question will inevitably be registered as "empty" without feedback. On the other hand, foci of inflammation and fungal nests can develop undisturbed.

The question naturally arises as to the cause of the fibre loss. In addition to the reasons already mentioned, another trigger comes into play: Nerves degenerate when they are not used, e.g. when the *receptors in the tissue are blocked*. Alkaloids are fungal toxins that are similar to hormones and are capable of these blockages.

*F. Boesser* already had good success with *antidotes*, e.g. ergot. But green tea extract also works in this direction, as does tannin.

Cholesterol infusions used to be used successfully. This makes sense because the alkaloids, which are similar in their structural formula, can be competitively displaced.

Before the era of antibiotics, cholesterol was also part of the therapeutic repertoire and was able to save lives because it is an important membrane component that protects cells from attacks.

The loss of afferent nerves is a serious barrier to healing and increases the risk of recurrence. To bridge the gap, the associated brain area should be supplied with the missing information using biofeedback.

The MRT 503 and the Equalizer EQ 103 are suitable for this purpose.

### 4.5.1. Archaic direct current system

In addition to the well-known complex nervous system, there is still the original form that can be found e.g. in amphibians. It is a direct current system that works via the *Schwann's* sheaths and forms a ***neural network***. The special thing about it is the polarity (forehead negative, neck positive), which can be reversed by the event of illness, so that the same therapy stimuli may be answered in the opposite way. A sleeping pill can then, for example, make you awake.

That's not all. This network forms maser holograms (in the microwave range) that depict all structures. These are practically the guide rails into which our cells grow and form organs. And here lies the problem at the same time.

Since these are microwaves that form interference, they can interfere with other microwaves (cell phone) and be significantly disrupted. Incidentally, this also applies to the EIEC described above.

In addition, Handy & Co. lead to de-myelination of the nerves and thus destroy the basis for these holograms. In this way, the cancer-promoting effects of technical radiation, but also geopathic fault zones, can be explained physically.

It is therefore imperative to do **without** these communication technologies.

### 4.6. Integration

Cancer means separation, breaking out of the existing order, loss of coherence and thus the cohesion of cells and tissues. In this context, however, the conditions that a living system needs for its maintenance and constant renewal are seldom discussed.

Matter alone is not able to generate life, even if it is tried again and again. The material components need a plan and a force to put them together. We know from quantum mechanics that matter can show intelligent behaviour. But how is that supposed to work with mindless building blocks?

Of course, it doesn't work without a controlling element in the background, and that is nothing other than our soul.

All activities of our organism, including cell metabolism, are an expression of the intelligently acting power of our soul, which acts as a mediator between spirit and matter.

The soul does nothing senseless. It pursues the divine plan set down in the spirit as an expression of higher consciousness. If we remove from it with our thoughts and actions, this will be tolerated for a short time.

Everyone may make mistakes. However, if the deviation gets bigger and bigger, we are warned with symptoms.

The next stage is then a disease (e.g. inflammation with a focal character). If there is no insight at all, the logical consequence is cancer at some point.

This philosophical view may not always be true because, as is well known, other reasons may also exist. But this makes the principle clear. We are spiritual beings; those of all creation (should) serve, but often enough not be able to withstand material temptations. And here a serious deficiency becomes clear: God's creation is a construct of love. We are flooded with it and can feel it when we go into resonance with it, e.g. in prayer or meditation.

## "Love is the force that holds the universe together." Prof H.P.Duerr

However, we can very easily disengage ourselves from this love by rejecting certain aspects of life. Nothing is bad per se.
It depends solely on our **judgment.** *René Egli* from Switzerland writes in his book 'The LoLa Principle': "All the misery on this earth begins with values and evaluations."

With the rejection of situations or certain people, we limit the radius of our soul more and more. According to the Hermetic Law, this affects our structure and function. What is not needed is receded. In this way we set off a development that after many years 'completely unexpectedly' can lead to cancer.

Without a loving approach to us and all of creation, health and well-being cannot be achieved in the long term. The cancer patient (and also every other chronically ill patient) has to come back there. And that is only possible by transforming all "negative" experiences and memories through a newly gained perspective. Conflict resolution and forgiving, dealing with all stressful events and returning to the quantum mechanical ground state is the main work that the patient has to do himself. Then a serious illness has fulfilled its purpose. That's the law.

### 4.7. Therapy concepts

Although in every chronic illness the loss of function of the basic regulatory system according to *Alfred Pischinger* – our matrix – is in the foreground, cancer differs from it in one essential point:

A cancer tumour can only develop if the **brain loses control** and the **holographic pattern of the maser radiation** that penetrates all cells and organs is disturbed.

The primary goal must therefore be to create the conditions for this again.

### A comprehensive therapy is therefore divided into

➤ Support of nerve regeneration and avoidance of damaging agents (cell phone, Wi-Fi, cordless telephone) to restore the maser hologram, which is essential for structure and order.

➤ Increase of the ionization energy through thyroid activation (thyroxine also promotes neurogenesis). The body temperature of 37° C (98.6° F) not only creates well-being, but is also a prerequisite for ATP production.

➤ Stimulation of the detoxification function and support of the kidneys, intestines and liver are a sine qua non, because the matrix burden could arise in the first place due to insufficient performance. Body heat also plays a role here.

➢ Initiation of a change in the patient's consciousness through education, acceptance of responsibility and self-love must not be neglected in any treatment. Otherwise we cannot speak of healing.

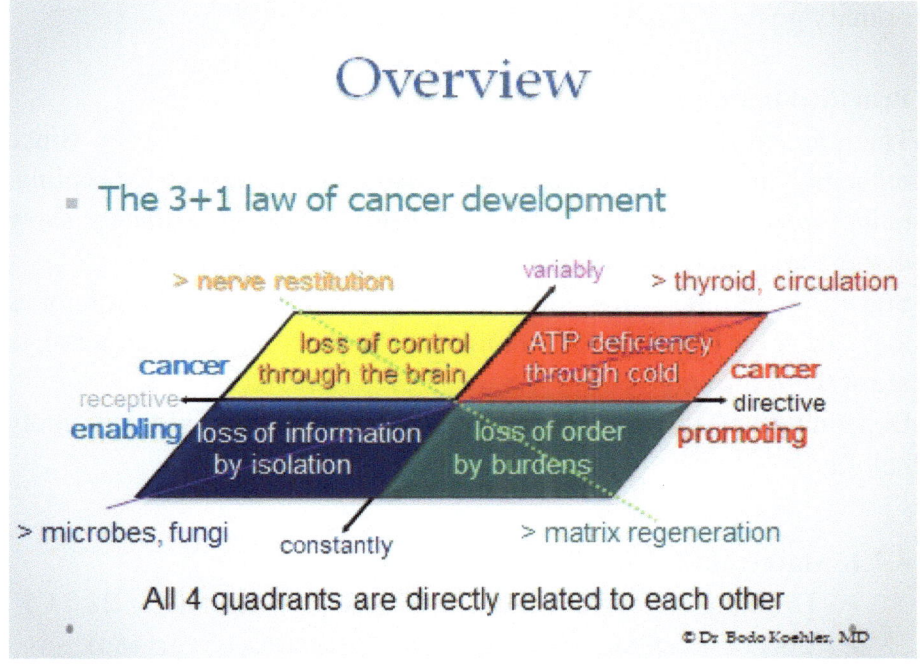

**Fig.11:** The main factors of carcinogenesis and measures

Cancer is curable, but not from outside. For this, the knowledge and conviction must be developed together with the patient. This is often tedious and often fails. Many patients are discouraged and have given up because they mostly only wanted to try "an alternative" in an advanced state. They are not to be blamed for that, as it is a problem of the lack of *comprehensive* oncological training of many colleagues.

The point is not at all to "remove" an unpleasant tumour, but to re-integrate the split off areas.

If it is possible to remove the tumour without causing additional harm to the patient, it can be very helpful in reducing anxiety, but it is not a primary goal.

**Practical implementation**
There are methods that work immediately; others take longer. Since reducing fear and building trust are essential prerequisites for healing, quick success is important. The well-being would immediately show that the treatment is working.
Since the multiple burdens of the matrix, together with the microbes that can never be neglected, are a heavy load, detoxification measures are at the forefront.
Depending on compliance, the following methods are extremely helpful:

**4.7.1. Matrix detoxification and cleansing**
- ➤ Drinking cure with approx. 4-5 l spring water daily (> 21 ° C)
- ➤ Lots of green tea, 10 minutes of boiled water (Ayurveda)
- ➤ **M**atrix **R**egeneration **T**herapy with MRT 503
- ➤ Connective tissue massages & lymph drainage (no contraind.!)
- ➤ LYMPHO*DYN*® and CMR / Vortex locally (tumour region)
- ➤ Elimination of foci with LSIT, procaine or surgically, e.g. teeth
- ➤ Kidney support (horsetail, goldenrod), CMR / Vortex
- ➤ Oil pulling through teeth, liver detoxification acc. to *Moritz*
- ➤ Enemas with organic Mexican highland coffee
- ➤ Colon hydrotherapy and intestinal symbionts, colostrum
- ➤ Procaine infusions (without added bicarbonate)
- ➤ Autologous blood therapy, HOT, high-dose ozone therapy

- *Baunscheidt* method, detoxification method acc. to *Aschner*
- Helpful: strong heat (hyperthermia, red light, sauna, hot bathes)
- Lugol's solution (HR → 120) with cardiac support (digitalis)
- Blood circulat.↑ drainage↑ (venous, lymph > LYMPHO*DYN*®)
- Light therapy (local laser, red light), red light laser i.v.
- pH shift with acids (citrus, vinegar) > alkaline
- Rectal ozone insufflation
- Balneotherapy (*Stanger, Kneipp*)
- Shorter or longer fasting (according to the constitution)
- Sweaty physical activity, hormesis
- Basic tone therapy acc. to Prof *V. Mukunda,*
- Sound bed, local sound application, local sound application
- Correct polarity of the DC system → NEC 708
- Coherent photons → CMR / Vortex, MRT, Equalizer EQ 103
- Electrons + protons → *Budwig* diet, MRT 503, EQ 103

The abbreviations listed are used to refer to the **Living Systems Infor**-**mation Therapy LSIT** (see literature; there exists a book in English with the same title).

These and other methods also serve to gradually exchange the body water with the stored pathological information, to balance the pH value in the tissue (standard 7.0) and to restore its day-night rhythm.

The success is shown in the urine: in the morning approx. pH 5, at noon 7, in the evening 5.
This has nothing to do with the tissue pH, but rather reflects the function of the liver. If the rhythm described above is correct, this is one of the prerequisites for the normal detoxification function. The rhythm can be supported by methionine (SAM-e) in the evening and potassium citrate in the morning. The dosage depends on the urine pH.

### 4.7.1.1. Breakdown of fungal toxins
- Fungi cannot be killed; they transform under stress
- Medicinal fungi (brewer's yeast! Reishi, Maitake, Chaga etc.)
- Avermectins (Ivermectin) "Scabioral", "Driponin"
- Fungi nosodes (acc. to testing)
- Neutralization of toxic alkaloids with cholesterol infusions
- High-dose vitamin C infusions
- Autologous blood therapy
- Plasmapheresis or apheresis
- Tannin, CurSiMag, *Secale cornutum D3*
- Acid substances: lemon puree (with peel), vinegar > basic
- Change in diet according to blood group;
- Carbohydrates↓ Omega oils↑ (krill oil)
- Coccidia: coffee enemas, colon hydrotherapy, local ozone
- Oregano, garlic, propolis, coconut oil, taraxacum
- Movement training
- *Sun!* → ionization energy

### 4.7.1.2. Adjuvant procedures
- Electro-therapy according to *Pekar / Nordenstroem*
- Local heat by radiotherapy (prostate)
- Hormones (breast & prostate) testosterone, progester., estriol
- ELDI oils according to *J. Budwig*, linseed oil quark diet
- Local laser therapy (metastases, Prof Dr *Vogel*, D-Frankfurt)
- *Gerson* therapy (Tijuana Mexico, vegetable juices, enemas)
- Leprosy model (CMR/Vortex, therapy with hereditary nosodes)
- *Banerji* homeopathy
- *Moritz* oil cure, oil pulling through teeth, oil enema (*Budwig*)
- Ayurveda
- Stem cell therapy (Dr *Nesselhut*), THX and PPX (thymus cure)
- Active fever therapy (with viruses, Dr *Thaller*, Germany)

> Basic tone therapy (acc. Prof *Vemu Mukunda*)
> Autonomy training (acc. Prof *Grosshardt-Maticek*)
> Laughter therapy
> Two animals passage (with cancer serum)

## 4.7.1.3. Preparations and food supplements

> Zeolite (KlinSiMag / CurSiMag)
> Proteolytic enzymes (f.e. Wobe-Mugos)
> Minerals and vitamins acc. test, MAP (amino acids pattern),
> α-lipoic acid, acetyl-carnitine, s-acetyl glutathione infusions
> Metformin, Tagamet
> Liver activation (silymarin, taraxacum, ornithine, Gelum)
> Nitrooxygen activation (arginine 4g in the evening.)
> Mistletoe, african frankincense
> Houttuynia, Takuna (antiviral for herpes, EBV, cytomegaly)
> Banderol, Samento (antibacterial for Borrelia, chlamydia)
> Nosodes of bacteria, viruses, vaccinations (acc. to testing)
> Resveratrol (red wine), astragalus
> Terpenes (essential oils e.g. lime, fennel, caraway, peppermint, rosemary), valerian, olives; ginkgo, cloves, birch bark; carotenoids, piperine (black pepper)
> Apple peel, gooseberry, blueberry (cooked), wild herbs, catechins (cocoa, green tea)
> Iodine, selenium, zinc, magnesium, tyrosine (see section 4.7.3)
> Heart strengthening with glycosides, hawthorn, Q 10, NADH
> Melatonin high dose (20 mg), 5-HTP, SAM-e
> Glucosa-K2 (epiphyseal decalcification, matrix renewal)
> *Bach* flowers, low dose naltrexone (schizophrenia, addiction)
> Peroxodisulfuric acid (strongly diluted, 3 tsp. daily) radicals ↑

This special sulfuric acid ($H_2S_2O_8$) stimulates the formation of radicals in the tumour cell, which promotes differentiation.

This list is by no means complete. A few more aspects will be added later. Above all, food for thought should be given. But it cannot be repeated often enough: First or in parallel, but never last, the milieu should be rehabilitated and the causes responsible for it eliminated!

In order to make life difficult for the parasites in a targeted manner and to bring back lost ground, the recommended measures according to Chapter 4.7.3. strongly advised.

At the same time, since a longer lead time is to be expected, the restitution of the maser hologram, which is necessary for the structure construction, takes place. Non-negotiable, however, is the ***total renunciation of cell phones & Co.*** (including Wi-Fi and cordless telephones). The selection is based on the possibilities in practice.

## 4.7.2. Nerve restitution

➢ Geopathic rehabilitation of the sleeping area
➢ 7-9 hours of sleep, darkened, reduced noise, 18 ° C room temp.
➢ DC polarity reversal with NEC 708
➢ Biofeedback with the brain (MRT 503, Equalizer EQ 103)
➢ Direct current pulsing (LYMPHO*DYN*®), *Schumann* frequency
➢ Detox of amalgam, cadmium, lead, aluminium
➢ Elimination of vaccination damage (with LSIT), environmental toxins (dioxin!)
➢ Neural therapy, procaine infusions (without bicarbonate)
➢ Transverse flow of the brain (short wave acc. to *Schliephake*), CMR / Vortex
➢ B vitamins + uridine monophosphate (Keltican forte)
➢ Parthenolide (feverfew), α-lipoic acid, acetyl-l-carnithine
➢ Phosphatidyl serine, omega 3 oils (krill oil or linseed oil)
➢ Ketogenic diet, coconut fat, oil pulling through teeth
➢ Coherent light (laser), red light (630 nm)

> ➢ Organ therapy (WALA, Regeneresen)
> ➢ Music (also as *Haffelder* CD), singing, humming in keynote
> ➢ Regular sexual intercourse, laughter therapy
> ➢ Walks in the woods and lots of sun, aroma therapy
> ➢ Stimulation of the thyroid gland see Chap. 4.7.3

All measures are dependent on the normal functioning of the metabolism of all cells. A prerequisite for this is a **balanced diet with greatly reduced carbohydrate** intake, geared towards the blood group. The thyroid gland plays a special role in the 4-pole regulation of cell metabolism according to *J. Schole* (Fig. 1). It is also responsible for ensuring that the **ionization energy** is sufficiently high. It therefore depends on it how many free charge carriers (ions, electrons and protons) are available. The food components can only be processed in the ionized form. Otherwise there will be deficiencies.

The other important aspect is the dependency on the venous blood flow and lymph, so that local stasis does not occur. These can prepare the ground for parasites, particularly fungi.

### 4.7.3. Activation of the thyroid function
> ➢ Brown algae (Kelp, Ecklonia cava) high dose
> ➢ Lugol's solution (HR → 120) with cardiac support (digitalis)
> ➢ Selenium (300-900 µg) morning, zinc (80 mg) in the evening
> ➢ L-tyrosine (→ dopamine, thyroxine)
> ➢ Magnesium (300-600 mg)
> ➢ Thyroxine substitution (if blood tests require it; TSH > 1)
> ➢ Compensate for progesterone deficits based on blood findings
> ➢ Breakdown of antibodies via autologous blood therapy
> ➢ Organ therapy (Regeneresen, WALA)
> ➢ Local neural therapy (2x1 ml 1% procain both sides)
> ➢ Liver support (breakdown pathway T4 > T3)

Life is not worth staying without meaning and purpose. Cancer is the external characteristic of *giving up on oneself*. A longing for death is projected into the future.

No cure can occur under these circumstances. "Enthusiasm for life" is polar opposite to self-abandonment. This "spin flip" has to be worked towards in many one-on-one discussions.

### 4.7.4. Shift in consciousness
- ➤ Conflict resolution, forgiving (mother and father!)
- ➤ Processing of the triggering event, mostly loss
- ➤ Shock resolution (CMR/Vortex, MRT 503, Equalizer EQ 103)
- ➤ Patient should be committed to the truth, not lies
- ➤ Implementation of suppressed needs of the soul, new relations!
- ➤ Family, friends, job, hobby, atmosphere…
- ➤ Apartment, place of residence, country versus city...
- ➤ New meaningful tasks
- ➤ Understanding the illness as a learning task
- ➤ Taking responsibility for life, learning self-love
- ➤ From the taker to the servant consciousness
- ➤ Consciously seek out the quantum mechanical ground state
- ➤ Meditation, autogenic training
- ➤ Food for the soul: poetry, music, painting, nature experiences
- ➤ Flavours, colours, walks in the woods
- ➤ Understand yourself as an indispensable part of God's creation
  Compare also Chapter 3.9.2. "Realignment" on page 83.

As explained in previous chapters, the tumour itself is only used as a *reference* to document the progress of therapy. This is not always possible, as it is not uncommon for patients to decide on naturopathic treatment only after an operation. Then there are other parameters, e.g. tumour markers.

In addition, if the location is favourable, experienced cancer specialists can certainly attempt to infiltrate the tumour with bicarbonate, while at the same time inhibiting carbonic anhydrase with acetazolamide. The same applies to the Galvano therapy according to *Pekar / Nordenstroem*.

After studying the literature as well as his own experience, *W. Zoech* suggests the following for local tumour treatment (quote):

"In principle, therapy is quite simple by offering the cancer cells large amounts of **bicarbonate**[1], which they "greedily" import and at the same time block **carbonic anhydrase**[2], which leads to a brilliant increase in intracellular carbonic acid. Bicarbonate supply leads to acidification (sic!) if carbonic anhydrase (acetazolamide "Diamox") is overstrained or inhibited, because the non-decomposing carbonic acid dissociatively adjusts itself to a pH value around 6.5. The cancer cell dies of carbon dioxide poisoning."

Reference:
1) Robey IF, Baggett BK, Kirkpatrick ND, Roe DJ, Dosescu J, Sloane BF, Hashim AI, Morse DL, Raghunand N, Gatenby RA, Gillies RJ "Bicarbonate Increases Tumour pH and Inhibits Spontaneous Metastases" Abstract quote "... This treatment regimen was shown to significantly increase the extracellular pH, but not the intracellular pH, of tumours by 31P magnetic resonance spectroscopy and the export of acid from growing tumours by fluorescence microscopy of tumours grown in window chambers...." Cancer Res 2009; 69: (6): 2260-8, March 15, 2009

2) Xue-Jun Li, Yang Xiang, Bing Ma and Xiao-Qiang Qi "Effects of Acetazolamide Combined with or without NaHCO3 on Suppressing Neoplasm Growth, Metastasis and Aquaporin-1 (AQP1) Protein Expression" Int. J. Mol. Sci. 2007, 8, 229-240, March 13, 2007

### 4.7.5. Dissolving the acid mantle of the tumour

- ➢ Injection of bicarbonate locally (!)
- ➢ Carbonic anhydrase inhibitor (e.g. Diamox – cave Pot.↓)
- ➢ Balancing the electron distribution (using LSIT)
- ➢ *Original* Gelum drops (lactate – acc. to Dr *Fryda*) → butyrate
- ➢ Procaine infusions with magnesium citrate (without bicarbon.)

The local bicarbonate injection is very promising for tumours that are not too deep. It already has been used often in connection with acetazolamide systemically. But despite everything, the basic problem is not solved, namely the ***cell milieu poisoning***, which is ultimately also responsible for the loss of control by the brain.

But every measure that can be carried out here with relatively little effort and few side effects creates hope and trust. Under no circumstances should it be left at that! This is because the cause was not recorded, and recurrences must be expected.

Therefore, a selection from the four mentioned points is still necessary in order to tackle the problem at the root. Only then can a real cure be achieved and indeed: cancer is curable!

Priority is given to detoxification and treatment of the causes. They consist in conflict resolution and transcendence of the triggering event.
Tolerance turned into weakness with intolerance towards oneself, thereby self-deception, self-lies, inconsistency result. Important decisions were not made, up to and including self-abandonment. The connection to the present was completely absent.

Only when the higher sense is understood can healing happen.

## Findings

*Everyone is a distinctive individual and, in the event of illness, also needs therapy that is tailored to them as precisely as possible.*

*There are therefore many starting points that must be taken into account. This can be confusing at first, which is why it cannot be dealt with in a target-oriented manner without a hierarchy. However, there are some points that practically always come into play and may never be neglected.*

*This includes **body temperature**, for which the thyroid is primarily responsible. Very many people have a disorder in this important organ, but they do not know it. Here prophylactic measures could already be taken.*

*Another point is the **circulation**, especially in the microscopic small capillaries (microcirculation) and the fine lymph vessels.*

*Here in particular, flow disturbances often occur, which can prepare the ground for **parasites**. These are mainly responsible for the loss of vital information, especially for the differentiation of stem cells.*

*The human being is a highly tensioned **electrical system**. All body functions are based on this. The most important charge carriers (besides the ions) are the **electrons** (deacidifying, carriers of experience), as opponents to the protons, which acidify the tissue. These relationships are in the foreground. Nevertheless, they are not taken into account in a conventional medical practice.*

*The formation of the **maser hologram**, which is formed by the archaic nervous system and represents the template for all forms (organs, etc.), depends on the electrical voltage.*

*The nerve function is also electrical, just as the regression of nerve fibers is related to a **loss of tension**.*

*The **milieu** in the family and at work (context) should not be underestimated. Every disease, but also healing process, is very strongly influenced by it. Stress often has deep roots that extend into **childhood**. Above all, the **mother and / or father relationship** plays a decisive role. Many tensions and conflicts in life can be attributed to it.*

*These can materialize as interference fields. Psych trauma, chronic inflammation, heavy metal pollution and parasitosis are usually connected, which requires a comprehensive therapy concept.*

*During the diagnosis, all of these points should be clarified and then a targeted selection should be made from the treatment proposals given. Nothing should be neglected!*

*The **dissolution of the tumor** is a great success. But it only serves the patient's peace of mind. It has nothing to do with healing yet. This should have been understood at this point at the latest.*

# 5. Prevention and diagnostics

The best cancer treatment is one that can be done without. Therefore, prevention should and can be done whenever possible. Amazingly, cancer has a lot to do with inflammation.

Inflammation (not infection), on the other hand, has a lot in common with aging processes. Prevention therefore not only means prophylaxis, but also more vitality. That is why inflammation is the focus.

## 5.1. The consequences of chronic inflammation
➢ Standstill of cell regeneration (anabolic derailment)
➢ Overstimulation of growth factors > risk of cancer"
➢ Increased formation of new blood vessels
➢ Senescent fibroblasts activate EMT > cancer risk↑
➢ Destruction of the extracellular matrix by metalloproteinases
➢ Activation anabolic hormone receptors (estrogenic dominance)
➢ Lack of DNA repair, mitochondria mutation
➢ *Warburg* effect (anaerobic glycolysis), activation of telomerase

## 5.2. Overcoming chronic inflammation
➢ Strengthen function of pituitary, thyroid and adrenal gland
➢ Balancing cell metabolism with CMR / Vortex, MRT, EQ 103
➢ Restoring of the microbiome! ("Effective Microorganisms")
➢ Adapted exercise (in the forest!), sports, sun
➢ Omega 3 oils, lecithin > krill oil! Potassium, vitamins B1, B6,
➢ Support with curcumin (CSM), resveratrol, piperine,
➢ Frankincense (Boswellia), proteolytic enzymes), 25mg Aspirin
➢ Amino acid l-carnosine against AGEs and toxic metals
➢ Heat (red light), hyperthermia, active fever therapy
➢ Ozone therapy, HOT, autologous blood, autologous urine

A special form are auto-immune diseases in which tolerance training of the thymus has failed. But that can be made up for.

## 5.3. Causes for the triggering of auto-immune disorders

- Lack of sun, more common in the north
- Lack of exercise, lack of forest walks!
- Anabolic or catabolic derailments
- Nitro oxygen deficiency, reduced detox capacity (lymph, liver)
- Burdens of foci, metal residues, calcifications
- Increase in NF-kappaB due to multiple stimuli
- Delayed healing processes
- Milk consumption! (B9 receptor block)
- Receptor blockages by bacteria / viruses
- "Vitamin" D supplementation for VDR blockade
- Lectins (in vegetables) can cause autoimmune diseases

Healing inflammations often mistaken for infection and treated with antibiotics. This is an absolute contraindication!

## 5.4. Useful diagnostics
In addition to the usual orthodox medical diagnostics, there are some key points that should definitely be taken into account:

- When and under what circumstances (context) did "desire for life" become no-desire with denial of desire-full needs?
- Which loss of relationship was responsible for this?
- For whom was she/he a substitute > mother or father?
- Thorough clarification of mother/father relationship > childhood
- Permanent burdens from negative person / object > helpless
- Personal environment, life styles, addictions, dependencies
- History of stress and shock situations
- Luescher test, classification in the Luescher cube
- EEG according to *Guenter Haffelder* > music CD
- Ability to regulate the cell metabolism CM (CMR, MORA*nova*)
- Functional examination of the 3 hormonal glands of cellmetab.

- Thyroid diagnostics, selenium, zinc, progesterone
- Milieu check (electro smog, geopathy)
- Test for vaccine damage
- Test for environmental toxins (Bisphenol A, dioxin, PCP)
- Test for pesticides (Glyphosate, DDT)
- Test for heavy metals (lead, mercury, Cd, Pd, arsenic)
- Ti, Ni, aluminium (promotes the spread of Borrelia & viruses)
- Neurotoxic viruses: Cytomegaly, EBV, varicella, HHV VI
- Enteroviruses: polio, coxsackie, echoviruses
- Enterobacteria: yersinia, enterobacter, campylobacter
- Borrelia; chlamydia, mycoplasma, legionella
- Fungi, coccidia
- LPS (endotoxins using the Limulus amoebocyte lysate test)
- Foci diagnostics (DFM, VEGA-Check, decoder, kinesiology)
- Eating habits, blood group (relation omega-oils to proteins)
- Stool sample (detox performance), bile acids, leaky gut
- Sedimentation rate, blood count, CRP, cholesterol, NF-kappaB
- Electrophoresis, IGF-1 (inflammation, protein deficiency)
- Blood sugar profile + insulin, HbA1c, triglycerides (diabetes)
- Thyroid parameters, Se, Zn, progesterone
- Liver values, kidney function, AB determination, TU markers
- Urine test: 3-fold pH measurements (liver function)
- Nagalase (as an indication for therapy with GcMAF)
- Sex hormones, pregnenolol, DHEAS, Estronex test
- Receptor status > representing 'vitamin" D receptor
- B vitamins (stomach acid deficiency?)
- Autonomic nervous system (HRV, tonometry) +/- polarity
- Neuromodulators (in saliva)
- Beliefs (Kinesiology)

Mammography and puncture should be avoided (risk of cell spread).

## 5.5. Strengthening the immune system

- Astragalus membranaceus (China)
- Beta-Glucan (brown algae), AHCC (mushroom extract) beer yeast
- Butylated hydroxytoluene BHT (preservative)
- "Opium" salad (chicory, radicchio, endive, lettuce, basil, hops!)
- Cordyceps sinensis (Chinese caterpillar fungus)
- Lithium (calms, supports immune system & promotes regener.)
- Indium (massively improves the absorption of nutrients)
- Blood transfusion (fresh blood)
- Korean ginseng
- Taiga root (eleutherococcus)
- Cocoa (only roasted at 115 °)
- Cannabis! Ashwaganda
- GABA (steamed tomato, potato, sprouted rice)
- Mucuna pruriens (pruritus bean, stimulates dopamine synthesis)
- Gotu kola (centella asiatica, "herb of enlightenment")
- Acetyl-l-carnitine together with alpha-lipoic acid
- Krill oil

God's pharmacy offers us a rich selection of helpful substances:

## 5.5.1. The most important herbal medicinal substances

- Resveratrol (red grapes, peanuts, currants, plums, tomato peels)
- Pterostilbens (=double methyl. resveratrol, dark berries, garlic)
- Curcuma (600 indications, NF-kappaB↓ diabetes↓ Alzh.↓ inflammatory↓ fats↓ AGEs↓)
- Terpenes (essential oils e.g. lime, fennel, caraway, peppermint) > tumor elimination!
  - Mono-terpenes: valerian, olives;
  - Di-terpenes: Taxol, rosemary, ginkgo
  - Tri-terpenes: olives, cloves, mistletoe, birch bark
  - Tetra-terpenes: carotenoids

> ➤ Fisetin (apples, gooseberry: stabilizes resveratrol; activates regeneration, antitumor effects)
> ➤ Piperine (black pepper: improves bioavailability)
> ➤ Putrescine from ornithine > spermidine, spermine

Several of these natural substances should be on the menu every day, not just pepper. However, it is better to use it consciously without stress in the kitchen, combined with gratitude for these gifts from nature.

**Natural Resveratrol Sources**
> ➤ **Vegetables:** cress, artichokes, asparagus, leafy vegetables, all kinds of cabbage, peppers, wild carrots, celery, cucumber, spinach, pumpkin, zucchini, eggplant
> ➤ **Fruit:** citrus fruits, olives, apples, strawberries, plums, figs, raspberries, pears, melons, currants, grapes, cooked blueberries (cooked!)
> ➤ **Herbs:** basil, rosemary, thyme, parsley, sage, dandelion, hawthorn berries, plantain, mint, rose hip, chamomile, milk thistle, lemon verbena, chilli

**5.6. Living Systems Information Therapy LSIT**
> ➤ Chakra therapy (synchronizing with quantum space, stress reduct.)
> ➤ Meridian therapy, wrist electrodes (soul connection)
> ➤ Basic tone therapy (harmony with orig. information, deceleration)
> ➤ Matrix Regeneration Therapy MRT 503 1x / week (burden↓)
> ➤ Local foci treatment (MRT, CMR / Vortex, Equalizer EQ 103)
> ➤ Cleaning of the receiving channel with Equalizer EQ 103
> ➤ Sympathetic-parasympathetic balance with Equalizer EQ 103
> ➤ Biofeedback with the brain (MRT 503, Equalizer EQ 103)
> ➤ Drainage therapy (vaccinations, toxic metals)
> ➤ Constitution therapy (coherence module, colours, basic tone)

➢ Polarity reversal, vegetative rhythm therapy with headphones
➢ Coherence therapy, respiratory therapy (rhythmiz. of the heart)
➢ Radiating the tumour information in the brain (feedback)
➢ Autologous blood, urine (microbes and LPS)

## 5.7. Special diet according to J. Schole
➢ Strictly avoid the following carbohydrates for 6 weeks:
  o Grains (rice, corn, wheat, rye, etc.)
  o Sugar (all sweets, honey), sweet fruits
  o Cooked root vegetables (carrots etc.)
  o Beer, spirits

**Effects:**
➢ Increased production of ketones > basic nutrition for the brain!
➢ Degradation of **AGE**s (**A**dvanced **G**lycation **E**nd products)
➢ M. Alzheimer's and dementia are on the decline
➢ Fatty liver (NAFLD) is regressing
➢ Insulin resistance is eliminated > risk of diabetes decreases
➢ Atherosclerotic plaques are broken down
➢ Tumour risk drops dramatically
➢ HGH increases
  o weight loss
  o muscle building
  o regeneration
  o enhancement of the immune system
  o dissolution of foci of inflammation

These effects already appear after 6 weeks, which is why this type of diet change is the most effective, not only for cancer patients. The older the patient, the slower the changeover!

In addition to the above limitation, there are the following ***contraindications:***

112

Sarcoid (M. *Boeck*), liver cirrhosis, seropositive rheumatism.

In all chronic diseases there is a derailment of the cell metabolism; either anabolic or catabolic (see Fig. 1, page 16). That is an absolute obstacle to healing! The main reasons for this are permanent psychological stress (fear!) and blockade of the HGH-releasing factor by insulin. This ketogenic special diet according to *Schole* alone enables cell metabolism to normalize!


**Findings**

*Cancer is a complex problem, but one that has clear principles. The accumulation with increasing age underlines the previous statements. Because year after year, the connective tissue matrix is more stressed, with simultaneous disruption of the lymph drainage.*

*The organism's often laborious attempt to rid the tissues of their burden through inflammation not infrequently becomes a chronic process.*

*This is not least due to the lack of ionization energy and the loss of control of the brain due to nerve degeneration.*

*Direct sunlight, which is usually avoided for fear of cancer, has a completely underestimated influence. But it protects against up to 17 types of cancer! The production of the D-hormone ("vitamin" D) is only a desired side effect.*

*It is not just sun heat that is responsible for protecting against cancer, but also UV rays in particular, which make life difficult for parasites.*

*Parasites play a major role in the development of cancer, but they are not the cause, but only the consequence of the loss of voltage (dielectric) in the matrix due to its various loads.*

*Therapeutic measures from nature can provide very good support.*

*Bioenergetic methods and special diets (Budwig, Schole) have a special position here.*

# 6. General overview

The attentive reader who has got this far will probably has a headache. So much data, so many facts! The fog can only clear if the main topic is kept in the foreground:

Cancer is the result of loss of control by the brain due to **neuro-degeneration** because of toxic matrix overload.

If it is possible to restore the full function of the CNS, the subject of "cancer" would be settled shortly with a few accompanying measures. But now, of all times, the viewer becomes unsure because this topic has not received any attention until now, yes, because this disease has been viewed from a completely different perspective, namely purely related to the tumour.

What does it mean to make the CNS fully functional again? That implies two things: First of all, it is about the restitution of degenerated nerve fibres. This primarily relates to the tumour area. But at the same time it affects the *neural function model*. The entire neural network generates a maser hologram, with which the tissue structure is determined and ordered. Missing nerves therefore lead to a defect in the hologram, which opens up space for chaotic structures.

A fully developed and functional nervous system completely rules out cancer!

That is the core message. The reasons for neurodegeneration have been dealt with extensively in this book (from Chapter 3.2, p. 62). Now it is a matter of making reconstruction possible and supporting it with targeted measures, but at the same time eliminating everything that prevents it (see Chapter 4.7.1. page 96). This includes, above all, all blockages that have been set by oneself.

What was initially useful as a protection against greater damage has a massive disease-promoting effect if the triggering event is not worked through and instead is permanently suppressed with high energy expenditure (consumption of essence electrons).

## 6.1. Neural network

Fortunately, nerve fibres can regenerate in opposite to earlier beliefs if the conditions are met. These include the ***building materials*** cholesterol (also formed in the brain), phosphatidyl serine, B vitamins and omega oils (e.g. krill oil or linseed oil).

An indispensable requirement is the ***normalization of the cell metabolism***, which is regulated by HGH (growth hormone) and the anabolic peptides for the synthesis metabolism as well as cortisol and thyroxine for the energy metabolism (Fig. 1 page 16). Thyroxine stands out because it is responsible for the necessary body warmth, but also promotes neuro regeneration. Special attention must therefore be paid to the thyroid gland (TSH should be around 1 (see Chap. 4.7.3. page 101).

This complex, highly dynamic interaction of the four regulators can only be influenced from the outside with ***Living-Systems-Information Therapy***. The CMR / Vortex and MRT 503 devices are suitable for this, but also the new Equalizer EQ 103 (Chapter 5.6. page 111).

But without these devices, an attempt should at least be made to record the current metabolic situation. Cancer always means catabolic derailment, which prevents cell differentiation. According to the laws drawn up by Prof *Juergen Schole*, supportive action must be taken here (read in "Regulatory Diseases" by *Schole / Lutz*, or in "Basics of Life" by *B. Koehler*).

Organ preparations, especially REGENERESEN (Dyckerhoff), but also fresh cells, have proven to be very effective. WALA manufactures homeopathic organ preparations, which are also well suited.

Neurogenesis can be started by stimulating all five senses. That is why music (also as *Haffelder* CD) and singing or humming in the keynote (personal basic tone) is very helpful, as are aroma therapy and walks in the woods.

Complete restoration of nerve fibres can take up to six months. Accompanying measures are therefore required to bridge the distance.

## 6.2. Biofeedback
Ultimately, it is about re-enabling the control function through the brain. This requires feedback from all body regions. This can be done using the above-mentioned LSIT devices in the same session, which makes treatment much easier. In the beginning this should be done once a week and later less and less as the well-being improves.

## 6.3. Accompanying measures
This includes all the registers that can be used for *matrix detoxification* (see Chap. 4.7.1. page 96). The focus is on *lymph flow*. Despite contradicting claims, lymphatic drainage is *not contraindicated* in cancer because the cancer model of conventional medicine is wrong. The feared sowing of cancer stem cells has long since taken place. However, these cannot grow under the observation of a fully functional brain – no chance!

Skilfully performed, regular *lymph drainage* is just as much a part of the program as the treatment with the newly developed **LYMPHO-**

*DYN®* **device**, which pushes the lymph in front via inductive direct current waves. But that's not all. The semiconductor effect of the silica-containing matrix is thus also increased, which results in an improved electron flow. But also the oxygen uptake and utilisation is improved with the device.

Again with information therapy, the tested (!) ***burdens of the matrix*** are drained individually – from vaccine damage to home toxins, aluminum and heavy metals, up to viral and bacterial colonisations. Special attention is paid to the ***fungi*** (diagnostics according to Chap. 5.4. page 108).

These measures not only support cancer treatment, but also have a preventive effect and slow down aging.

Basically, it can be said that ***bacterial infections*** rarely heal completely because fragments of them are usually left behind (lipopoly-saccharides LPS), especially after antibiotic treatment. These residues can stress the matrix for a lifetime, mainly because they are informative on the one hand and interfere with the dielectric on the other (matrix as electron storage). So if old infections appear in the resonance test, they should still be eliminated years later. Information therapy with nosodes or autologous blood treatment are suitable for this.

***Creeping infections*** (silent inflammation) must be decoupled from this. There is no victory for the immune system. Some of the microbes survive, especially in regions with poor blood supply with impaired lymph drainage, or intracellularly. Depending on the stress level (also dietary, e.g. sugar), these microbes can become active again.

This is especially true for *silent foci*, especially in the tooth and jaw area. These regions are critical because the microbes' toxins can easily penetrate the brain.

Antibiotic treatment is usually pointless because the blood does not get to the place where it happened. The poor circulation protects the microbes. Local red light treatment can sometimes work wonders here. Long-term treatment with *natural antibiotics* can be carried out in parallel (at least 6 months). If the microbes are not known, *Banderol* or *Samento* are particularly suitable (especially for Borrelia and chlamydia), otherwise nosodes can be used.

What is true of bacteria is particularly true of *viruses*. No virus can be defeated by the defence system! Specific antibodies have to be provided for a lifetime in order to stand up to the challenge, which puts a permanent strain on the immune system. The best example is varicella. These viruses can reappear at an advanced age, then as the dreaded herpes zoster.

For this reason, every anamnestic information must be checked, on the one hand with antibody detection in the blood, on the other hand with resonance test (Biotensor, EAV, kinesiology, etc.). The drainage takes place as above.

In the case of particularly *resistant viruses* such as herpes, EBV or Cytomegalie, natural antivirals can also be used successfully, e.g. *Houttuynia* or *Takuna.*

Those who have worked their way up to this point therapeutically and have eliminated most of the burdens (over a period of weeks) can now devote themselves to *fungi and their toxins*. This chapter alone is a great challenge.

Fungi cannot be destroyed. They sometimes even survive house fires. The ***thorough renovation of the cell milieu*** alone provides advantages for the immune system. Therefore the above measures must be taken first.

Medicinal mushrooms (Reishi, Maitake, Shitake, Chaga, etc.), but also brewer's yeast, especially for candida, offer very good support. Fungal nosodes (acc. to testing) also make sense.

If it is not entirely clear which species it is, an experiment with Avermectine (Ivermectin) ***Scabioral***, ***Driponin*** can be made after prior testing.

## Sufficient body temperature is a basic requirement for healing processes, but also every application of heat has a supportive effect.

In addition to the "corpses" of microbes, mycotoxins represent a major problem, especially the alkaloids. These have a neurotoxic and even directly carcinogenic effect.

As under point 4.7. listed on page 94, various measures are effective. A selection must be made depending on the equipment in the clinic. Ideally, the individual procedures should be tested for resonance in order to avoid excessive reactions. *Arndt-Schulz's* rule still applies: Weak impulses fuel life force, medium impulses strengthen them, strong ones destroy them.

A good ***cooperation with the patients*** is essential. Just changing the diet can give you a very strong boost. That should be done comparing to the blood group (according to Dr *D'Adamo*).

Basically, quickly usable carbohydrates have to be reduced, but also fructose. Who exercises a lot, which is desirable, burns more carbohydrates. Outside there is also a greater chance of soaking up more sun. This increases the ionization energy.

Acidic substances are helpful, e.g. lemon puree (with peel), but also vinegar. Extensive recommendations, in particular from the plant garden, can be found under Chap. 5.5.1. on page 110.

All suggestions and methods have the goal of bringing about changes in consciousness, on all levels of BEING. By changing the cell milieu, microbes can conquer areas in the human body. But this is not a passive process; it is accompanied by a high level of intelligence. It even goes so far that microbes, including fungi, contact us in order to specifically influence our psyche. This is well known from Toxoplasma gondii. This is possible in the quantum state of DNA.

## Viruses, bacteria and fungi are by no means our enemies! They live according to the cosmic laws like us and look for harmony.

That is an essential point. If you fight against microbes, you make them aggressive. Strictly speaking, they are a parameter for the state of our matrix and thus the inner life requirements. They only have a chance with us when they are exposed to the usual suspects.

The milieu renovation is therefore exactly the right way to restore the lost balance and to refer the intruders to their places. These are usually our mucous membranes.

Respect for other forms of life, which are just as much a part of creation as ourselves, is decisive for our work. Peaceful coexistence is only possible in LOVE.

## 6.4. Suggestions

This book would make little sense without clear practical guidance. Against the background that mass only makes up the billionth part of reality and that our existence is almost exclusively determined by *interaction quanta*, information therapy and thus consciousness clearly come to the fore. Because cancer genesis itself is based on a loss of information, locally and generally through the loss of control of the brain.

This can be triggered by a wide variety of noxae, up to a psychotrauma. But all the individual factors can be summarized in one point: It is always a question of a loss of *information* and thus a loss of shape in the tissue, which we call a tumour.

As in Chap. 1.5.1. explained in detail, the innumerable light quanta (photons) that circle in the electron tori are responsible for this. All events are stored in them as memories, imprint themselves on the matter and give a new order. Usually, it is used to adapt the various tissues to changing requirements and to constantly reshape them. The fabric structure is therefore always the reflection of the environmental influences – both inside and outside.

This customization usually works perfectly smoothly. However, it looks completely different with the interference fields.
Due to the overlay (contamination) with the earlier traumatic experiences stored here, there is no normal remodelling, but at best a standstill with degeneration. However, if the stressful memories are too massive, this chaos can materialize directly as a clumsy tumour mass.

To make matters worse, the originally alkaline environment has now become a highly acidic one, which paralyzes the immune cells and prevents any self-healing.

The dissolution of the acidic tumour mantle therefore has priority. There is the direct route by means of bicarbonate infiltration, if the area can be easily reached with the syringe.
The second variant is much gentler and uses the alkalizing potential of the electrons. Either direct current is introduced (e.g. using the *Pekar / Nordenström* method) or a strong flow of electrons in the tissue is stimulated by magnetic field induction. This can be done with LYM-PHO*DYN*®.

At the same time (!) the supply of electrons should be secured. The Budwig oil-protein diet offers the best conditions for this, with strict avoidance of trans fats.
This should be combined with initially gentle but intensive tissue cleaning. Deposited, denatured fat-protein compounds (lipoproteins) can ideally be broken down with natural enzymes and thus made transportable for the lymph flow. Vegetable juices **fermented with lactic acid** are particularly suitable for this, especially beetroot juice (contains indispensable molybdenum), sauerkraut juice, Kanne bread drink, etc. 2-3 litres of which should be consumed per day. Further hydration can be done with pure spring water or as green tea.

Under no circumstances should the sunshine be missing, of course without sun "protective agents", but well-dosed for up to half an hour at noon and correspondingly longer in the afternoon.
If this is combined with moderate endurance exercise, a good foundation has already been created for the further treatment steps, e.g. the Living-Systems-Information-Therapy LSIT.

The first LSIT devices were built in 1975 and experience has been gained in countless practices since then. 45 years are plenty of time for rapid developments in electronics. That pays off today. In the meantime, the knowledge of body physiology has progressed much further, so that treatment successes can be expected that we could only dream of before.

But even readers who are not familiar with it have a fund here from which they can draw for the benefit of their affected patients – not only with cancer. Everyone who is chronically ill can benefit from the methods of Life-Supporting Medicine LSM (see textbook "UNITED life-supporting MEDICINE").

### 6.4.1. First contact

Usually the patients come to us directly from the oncologist, insecure and full of fear of infirmity and death. Quite often they were also given a (bad) prognosis.

No matter what stage they are in – healing is always possible! This is proven by the spontaneous healings. It has to be conveyed to them, however, which is not infrequently met with disbelief because they have completely different ideas about their illness and have been indoctrinated accordingly.

We cannot convince anyone with words. Actions must follow that can build trust and confidence. Therefore, through a thorough anamnesis, in which the worries and needs are given high priority, the feeling should be conveyed: This is the right place for me. All my problems are taken very seriously, without any time pressure.

However, it is essential to clarify and work through a childhood issue with the mother / father relationship. As Prof *Grossarth-Maticek* has explicitly worked out, the foundation for health or cancer can be laid here.

For the resolution of a parental conflict (mother: rejected blue in the Luescher test, father: rejected red) the following points are important:

> Understanding, forgiving (also oneself), gratitude.
> Revive the genetic connection with love *
> Work through all hurts with a trusted person. If no serious events can be identified, deep-seated fear blocks access to the subconscious – because cancer patients without psych trauma do not exist!
> The time should be recorded when life changed from desire to listlessness and since then all lustful needs have been actively (!) suppressed.

Parallel to this, the home should be examined by a geobiologist. This also includes electro smog.

It is crucial that the conversations are conducted with eye contact and deep empathy. Only then can patients be reassured that they can get healed and that we will help them to do so.

To do this, however, the "tooth" should be pulled right at the beginning to fight the disease because it is bad for him and has to go. We want to achieve *re-integration*, collective coherence. This only works with love for themselves and all (separated) parts of the body.

---

* Since everything takes place on a spiritual level (quantum space), this ritual also has an effect beyond the death of mother or father. However, it is crucial that it is done with fervor and triggers strong emotions. If the parent is still alive, it should be done before the next visit. Then the change in consciousness that has already set in can already be seen. Words are then mostly superfluous – only LOVE counts.

The ritual with the mother holds an enormous healing potential and should therefore be at the beginning. Through the genetic connection, the exchange of essence electrons takes place much more intensively.

The question about the new tasks and goals *after* the recovery process is complete should also not be missing. Because many patients do not expect a cure at all, but rather think of an accompanying treatment.

In order to avoid frustration, a kinesiological test should therefore be carried out right at the beginning to determine whether the inner willingness for healing is actually present. Very often this is not the case!

As explained in the individual chapters, there is very often an inner desire to die. These patients have given up on themselves. If this is overlooked and therefore not dealt with, any further attempt at treatment is pointless.

### 6.4.2. Treatment plan

With all our measures we initiate and support the healing process, but we do not *make* anyone healthy. As a doctor and therapist, one should get rid of this hubris. But we set the plan according to the possibilities that arise in practice.

It doesn't make sense to do as much as possible at the same time. Well-coordinated step therapy is much more effective.

This is why even small practices can work very successfully if causal therapy is sought. The goal is always – not only in cancer – to enable the supply environment for the cells and the higher-level control by the brain. However, one cannot act cautiously enough. Each therapeutic measure must be processed by the patient with a corresponding expenditure of energy. This is where most of the mistakes happen. Cancer is the final stage of years of development. The resources are used up!

Therefore, a gentle supply of heat is recommended at the beginning at home, either with an infrared sauna, if available, red light or warm baths. It should not be forgotten that it is a catabolic derailment, i.e. a sickness based on inner coldness. These measures alone are therefore felt to be very beneficial.

After appropriate diagnostics, deficiencies are filled – vitamins, minerals, amino acids. What can be regulated about a change in diet has priority.

It is to be expected that deficiencies exist on different levels – up to a lack of love. As much as possible should be changed and the patient should be actively involved in the healing process.

### 6.4.3. Information transfer

At this point, some therapy methods with devices used for this purpose are addressed. If you want to go deeper into the method, you can acquire the necessary knowledge from my book "Living Systems Information Therapy LSIT" (English language).

The first thing to do is to ***normalize the derailed cell metabolism*** locally in the tumour region or in diagnosed foci. The CMR device 703 (Cell & Milieu Revitalization) is suitable for this. This means that the information from the missing hormone regulators is transmitted deeply via a magnetic field. At the same time, the microcirculation is stimulated.

The effect can be increased if the CMR is used in conjunction with the Vortex 705 device and the NEC 708 headphones. As a result, polarity reversal of the archaic direct current system can take place at the same time.

These are very gentle procedures that do not put additional strain on the organism.

Balancing therapy with the Equalizer EQ 103 is just as gentle, but sustainable. It not only allows old injuries to be dealt with, but also relieves shock.

It is particularly important to provide the brain with the missing information about the tumour region (feedback), which can be done very easily with this device. Such treatment can initially be carried out daily, then less and less.

The MRT 503 device (Matrix Regeneration Therapy) is also suitable for this. But that's just a welcome side effect. The main area of application is the detoxification of the matrix, for which the built-in cupping massage is particularly helpful. Additional information that is necessary for detoxification (e.g. glutathione) is retrieved from analogue stored memories.

This treatment can be exhausting and is therefore not used at the beginning, but only when the condition improves.

An essential part of the treatment is also the elimination of the tested toxins and parasites with information therapy.

Right from the start, however, the LYMPHODYN® device is in use, with which, via a pulse-controlled, rhythmic direct current flow, not only the lymph drainage is improved, but also the electron transport in the matrix is stimulated and at the same time oxygen utilisation is activated (increasing the anabolic metabolism).

With this directly the tumour region is treated, which means that local deacidification can also be achieved. The current flow stimulates the nerves, which supports neurogenesis – the goal of our efforts.

### 6.4.4. Supportive measures

At this point, those remedies that are useful for nerve regeneration should be mentioned (Chap. 4.7.2. p. 100), i.e. B vitamins with uridine monophosphate (Keltican forte), parthenolides (feverfew), phosphatidyl serine, krill oil (or linseed oil), organ preparations and of course a normal thyroid function with sufficient thyroxine for re-myelination. Therefore iodine should not be missing. Correspondingly high dosage stimulates the circulation, which is very desirable.

First of all, this sets priorities. A further selection for general treatment can be made from the lists from page 94; it would be optimal to test them out beforehand.

In addition to LSIT, somewhat more intensive applications have proven successful, such as autologous blood treatment, HOT or ozone therapy. As a high-dose OHT method, it is quite aggressive, but is particularly effective in the case of parasite infestation.
The high-dose treatment with proteolytic enzymes, vitamin C and *cholesterol infusions (!),* local procaine or as an infusion (without bicarbonate) offer very good support.

The treatment of the entire gastrointestinal tract, taking into account the necessary acidity (pH 5.8-6.3), is an indispensable aid both for the liver, which is usually completely overloaded, and for the immune system located in the intestine. The targeted use of symbionts (based on stool findings) can be supported with colon hydrotherapy.
Breast cancer in women and prostate cancer in men have a special position. First of all, the Estronex test should be taken into account as an important indicator of the breakdown pathways of female hormones in the liver. It can, for example, show that the methylation is insufficient and must be supported (e.g. with SAM-e).

In addition, there are excellent options for treating both types of cancer with nature-identical hormones (estriol, progesterone, testosterone).

Each treatment plan can only be created individually. Then an optimum is achieved. But never forget: Everything is consciousness!

This could be a rough outline of a weekly plan for a practice or clinic that is modified accordingly. The more information therapy, the fewer drugs are required.

| destination | method | Mo | Tu | We | Th | Fr |
|---|---|:---:|:---:|:---:|:---:|:---:|
| TU region | LYMPHODYN | X | X | X | X | X |
| TU region | ZMR/Vortex<br>alternatively<br>MORA, BICOM<br>Vegaselect | | X | | | X |
| CNS polarity | NEC 708 | X | X | X | X | X |
| TU region<br>> brain | Equalizer EQ 103<br>**feedback**<br>MRT 503 | X | X | X | X | X |
| matrix<br>detoxification | MRT 503<br>1x / week | | | | X | |
| matrix<br>toxins<br>remove | Equalizer EQ 103<br>ZMR/Vortex<br>MRT 503<br>alternatively<br>MORA, BICOM<br>Vegaselect | X | X | X | X | X |
| TU region<br>CNS<br>matrix | procain infusions<br>HOT, ozon therapy<br>cholesterol infusions<br>hyperthermia<br>laser therapy i.v. | X<br><br><br>X | <br>X | <br><br>X | X<br><br><br>X | <br>X |

**Table 1:** Therapy variant for the initial intensive treatment

Our beliefs and intentions are as much a part of the therapy as the patient's fears and worries. Only together can something be brought to a successful conclusion. This requires constant empathic exchange, because healing happens in love. Sometimes feeling loved (again) is the only key.

The medication is put together individually, if possible with a resonance test. Preparations for nerve regeneration and, in this context, also for the thyroid (selenium, zinc, iodine, possibly progesterone) are mandatory.

Patients can apply heat themselves at home, e.g. red light and in the form of a lot of green tea.

### 6.4.5. Philosophical aspect

Everyone is also a philosopher, although only a few have consciously integrated this into their lives. Philosophy – the love of wisdom – is the roof under which we live. It gives us foresight.

At the end I would like to give the reader something that can open the door to a completely new dimension of thinking. It's about mushrooms.

Its origin goes back more than 2 billion years. They are not only the oldest living beings, but also those with the greatest experience in survival techniques. But not only that – they had enough time to spread over the entire (!) earth. There is hardly a place where they do not exist. They have created a complete underground network with which they communicate worldwide. They appear as **guardians** and **protectors**, because it is they who have created all the prerequisites and thus the basis of life to enable higher development. They are the rulers of the world. None of the new forms of life could develop without them and their help.

The mushroom network serves, among other things, to connect the roots of the trees and plants with which they live in symbiosis. They are thus also administrators and guardians of botany.

They provide nutrients and thus make the flora possible in the first place, especially in less fertile regions. Without mushrooms, our range of fruit and vegetables would look much leaner. Maybe it wouldn't even be there? But fungi also enrich the laid table with fine dairy products that would otherwise not be available. We couldn't enjoy some baked goods, beer or wine.

But that is only the basis for a completely different consideration: The electromagnetic fields of the mushrooms generate interference with the environment. They stamp their information on all edible natural products – but also on us! As soon as we leave the house, we enter fungi terrain. These fields envelop us like rising fog on a damp meadow.

Mushrooms have a stable basic oscillation like the fundamental in music. Could it therefore be that our biological home is fungi and that we are in constant interaction with them?

Would it be conceivable that illnesses are based on a communication disorder with them and that fungal infestation, with all its toxic consequences, is not just a sign of loss of vitality and creeping death? Because mushrooms follow their assignment in the blue quadrant (water element). They are constant-receptive, adapt to external conditions and are therefore integrative.

They ensure that we can eat and live. But they are at the same time profiteers from death, although they usually do not wait so long for it to be completed. This can be seen well in infested old trees.

Mushrooms span the polarity between vitality and death. This is unique. So-called medicinal mushrooms can support healing and bring death to others. Even so, it is the same genus of the eukaryotes.

Why shouldn't we try to better understand the intelligence of mushrooms? Why is brewer's yeast beneficial, but not Candida, even though it is also yeast?

In fact, we have to have fungus genes within us. If our organism oscillates harmoniously, fungi are helpful and can support us. They reflect the simplicity. Anyone who does not adhere to it leaves this stable basic oscillation and becomes susceptible to diseases. The water element that is not lived – our personal satisfaction, basic trust, maintaining relationships also maintain, but a mother's love – brings us out of balance. Then integration changes to separation with all the negative consequences.

Every focus of illness is a separation, an aspect that has not been lived and a loss of vitality. This can trigger harmful fungi. These shift into the (acid) earth element (green – see Fig. 1) and burden us.
The counterpart to the mushrooms with their extensive wickerwork is our nervous system, which also belongs to the water element and whose basic oscillation corresponds to the individual keynote. It is the "master" of the earth element (green), the place for harmful fungi.

As the first inhabitants, mushrooms had to adapt to the fundamental oscillation of the earth, which corresponds to tone G and is at 385 Hz. It is not surprising that it is the resonance frequency of our DNA.
Restoring the harmony with mushrooms would therefore be quite easy with the dual tone of tone G with the individual keynote. A sound bed

(for the fundamental tone) and a sound applicator for local treatment with the tone G are ideally suited for this purpose.

The Indian atomic physicist and music therapist Prof *Vemu Mukunda* has succeeded in initiating healing in cancer patients by singing the keynote. This underlines this conceptual approach.

Fungi seem to have the wrong place in our society. Living close to nature also means recognizing mushrooms as our ancestors and paying them the necessary attention. They not only prepared our existence, they also enable our continued existence. Without them we would not exist.

Defying fungi is the wrong approach. Perhaps they are currently fulfilling important tasks in us? Do we even call harmful fungi on the scene with our negative emotions? The earth element symbolizes our authenticity. How could this lost?

When and under what circumstances did a patient leave his path, was he deceived or manipulated and thereby lost his self-determination?

## 7. Epilogue

Cancer is curable! That cannot be stressed enough. However, a differrent therapeutic approach is required here, in contrast to chronic diseases. Cancer can be understood as the result of all stresses in the course of life – mentally and materially – that have manifested themselves as cell milieu poisoning and prepare the ground for parasites. Accordingly, everyone should get cancer at some point. The tip of the balance, however, is the loss of control by the brain as a result of toxic nerve damage. Certain viruses are responsible for this, mostly from the herpes group. This, in turn, can be preceded by vaccination damage. Everything together creates the conditions for cancer to develop at all.

But there is also another, essential reason: we can characterize interference fields better than encapsulated areas from previous, serious injuries that have not been dealt with. This is done to protect the entire system. However, it leads to a higher energy consumption of *essence electrons*. Neurodegeneration also occurs in these quasi-disused areas. What is not needed is receded.

Nerve degeneration and with it loss of control by the brain is a central point in the development of cancer and at the same time a considerable obstacle to healing.

Cancer would be preventable if it were constantly ensured that the detoxification functions of the lymph, liver, gall and intestine remained fully functional and that there was no overload due to improper nutrition, especially carbohydrates, trans fats or low quality of animal protein (pigs!). The loss of control by the brain is an even bigger problem, however. It decides on the beginning, the course and thus the prognosis.

If you are an interested person who deals new with cancer, you may get a queasy feeling when reading the many triggers. But that is not the intention of this book. Rather, I have shown viable paths that are cause for optimism. That is the message!

Of course, the advice should be taken seriously, but there is no need to panic. Cancer is not just a physical disease. All structures with their functions are ***constructs of consciousness***. Unfortunately, this is rarely taken into account. Spirit creates matter (involution). All BEING is a thought-quantum-field structure, triggered by emotions and can / has to be corrected also on this level. We create our own reality through our goals and intentions – diseases too!

Quantum research opens up completely new perspectives for us. There are very well-documented courses of cancer that work like miracles for us, but can be explained with quantum mechanics – spontaneous healing of patients in the end-stage, complete disappearance of large tumours overnight or completely unexpected twists in the course of the disease.
For this, the illness has to be transcended, i.e. raised to the spiritual level. Quantum researchers call this bottom-up.

In the spirit – to be equated with quantum space – the triggering event (shock, conflict, etc.) can be transformed in love (!) with an expanded consciousness and brought back to reality with a new meaning (top-down).
Matter can dissolve again through a so-called spin flip. Growth turns into regression. It doesn't have to be decided by random. We can act on it with our consciousness. That is why personal realignment is so crucial. If we completely detach our circling thoughts from a problem – it doesn't always have to be illness – and let ourselves be fascinated

by new tasks, a spin-flip can occur, completely detached and without any compulsion.

Healing, however, does not happen then because we want it that way, but by resonance with our new structure of consciousness – of LOVE.

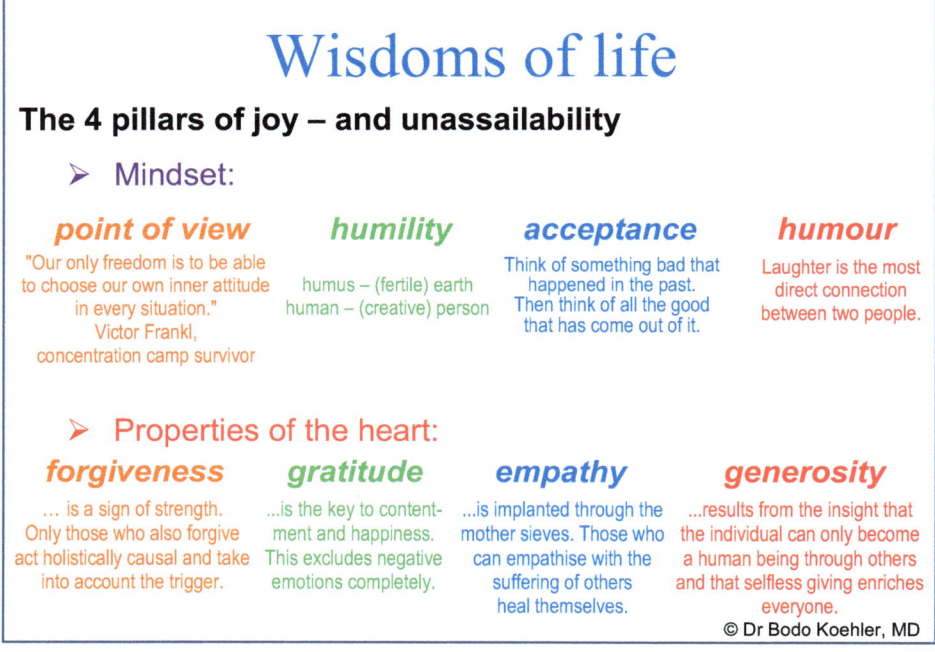

**Fig.12:** Those who manage to fully develop all 8 aspects of themselves will be able to lead a happy, fulfilled life (acc. to the "Book of Joy" by Dalai Lama, Desmond Tutu, Douglas C. Abrams)

In the infinite quantum space (spirit) there is an unlimited potential of possibilities that is just waiting to be called up by us. Then anything is possible. The limitation is made solely by our imagination. Limits are also set by the fact that many patients have already left life. Therefore a complete restart is necessary.

# List of figures

# *Bibliography*

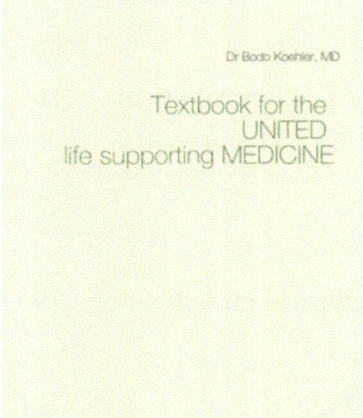

**Textbook for the UNITED life supporting MEDICINE** sets new accents in diagnosis and therapy of the chronically ill. It has put the research results of important scientists into practice and thus points the way for a long overdue combination of conventional medicine and naturopathy. This step leads into another dimension of medicine through the integration of synergistic methods. This results in a new quality, with which the long overdue paradigm shift can be initiated. Quantum physics has made a significant contribution to this and opened up new perspectives.

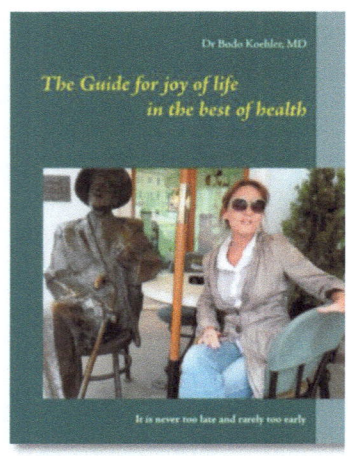

*The guide* deals with important everyday questions, starting with nutrition, through lifestyle, philosophical issues in life and medical problems, especially if they have arisen from the common errors of medicine. It is the author's concern to address and explain them openly, e.g. about civilization ailments such as arteriosclerosis, osteoporosis, etc. This book reflects extensive experience that has been gained in over 45 years of professional activity as an internist and doctor for naturopathic treatments. There is often a contrary perspective to the prevailing opinion, which can, however, be scientifically justified.

**Living Systems Information Therapy – Introduction to Quantum Medicine; Textbook for the medical and naturopathic practice**, 8th edition 2019, volumes I and II
This basic work describes the physically connections that are behind the phenomena of our reality.

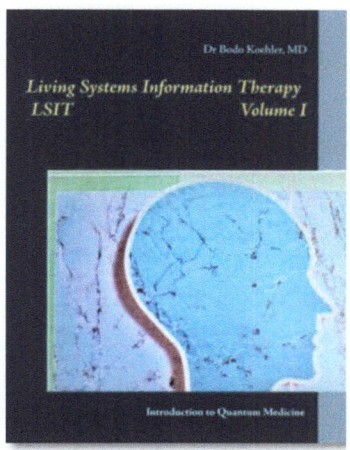

The Living Systems Information Therapy LSIT is able to initiate healing processes even in the case of advanced chronic diseases. For some indications, f.e. allergies, intoxications, etc., it is unsurpassed.
The textbook deals in detail and comprehensibly with the physical and biomedical basics of information therapy with internal and external signals as well as the "how" to use this form of therapy, which is increasingly popular, successfully and for the benefit of the patient.

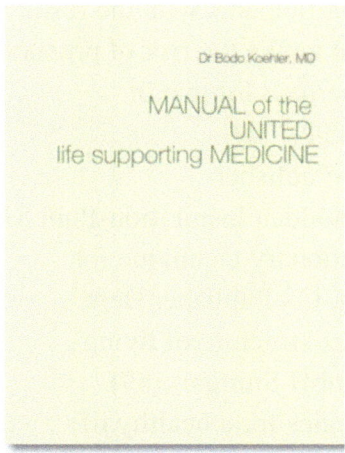

**MANUAL of the UNITED life supporting MEDICINE**
This manual is a short guide to get an overview of the complex contexts that are conveyed in the above textbook. In particular, the basics of life are brought into connection with the spiritual origin, which unfortunately is completely neglected in science. Only when the origin and function of living systems is understood can diseases be treated at the root and not just symptoms suppressed.

All these books can be ordered directly at **www.bod.de/buchshop**.

**Further literature sources:**
Abderhalden: The Abderhalden Reaction, Springer 1922
Becker, R.O.: Spark of Life, Scherz- Publisher München 1994
Boesser, F.: The solution to the cancer question, Hoffmann-
Publisher Barnstedt, 3. Edition 1985

Brandmeyer,
Koehler, B.: Light gives life, Publisher fit for Life
Bruker.M.O.,
Galtier: Cholesterol, the essential substance
Budwig, J.: The fat syndrome, Hyperion- Publisher Freiburg 1965
The elementary function of breathing... Hyperion-P.
Oil protein diet
The death of the tumour, volume II
Photo elements of life, Resch- Publisher
Cosmic power, Resch- Publisher
Being human, breathing, immune def. in a stranglehold

Chan, June
M. et al.: Long-term study on 21,000 participants with the result
that less than 600 mg calcium intake the risk of prostate
cancer increases by 32%.American Journal of
Clinical Nutrition 2001; 4: S.549-554
Charon, J. E.: The spirit of matter, Ullstein-Publisher
Death, where is your sting? Sudden Inspiration-Publ.81
Clark, R. H.: Healing is possible: A revolutionary technique for
treatment of chronic diseases, C.- Publisher Bern
Cramer F.: Chaos and order. The complex structure of living
Deutsche Verlags-Anstalt GmbH Stuttgart (89)
D'Adamo, P.: The 4 blood groups – 4 strategies for a healthy life
kindle edition
Dalai Lama, Desmond Tutu,
Abrams,D.C.: The book of Joy, Lotus-Publisher

Davidov,A.S.: Biology and Quantum Mechanics, Pergamon Press, Oxford 1982

Diefenb.,E.: Acids-base household, digestion & physiolog. flora

Dorandt,I.E.: Life in the fog

Droescher, W.

Heim. B.: Structures of the physical world and its non-materiel side, Resch-Verlag 1996

Duerr, H.-P.: There is no matter! Rotana-Publisher 2012

Eberhard, L.: Healing powers of colours, Drei-Eichen- Publisher, Munich 1954

Egli, R.: The LoLa principle, Editions d'Olt, CH-Oetwil
Illusion or reality? Editions d'Olt, Ch-Oetwil 2000

Endler, P.: Water and information, Allg. Homöopath. Zeitung 24.

Evertz, U.,

Koenig, H.L.: Pulsating magnetic fields in its meaning for medicine Hippokrates 48, 16-37, 1977

Evertz,U.,

Ludwig, W.: Magnetic field treatment, Frontier areas of science 26, 106-119, 1977

Frankl, V. E.: The human being faced with the question of meaning, Springer-Publisher 1979

Froehlich, H.: Biological coherence and response to external stimuli, Springer- Publisher 1988.
Interactions of non-linear wave mechanisms between excitable tissue and electromagnetic fields, Neurol.Res. 1982, 4 (1-2), p 115-153, ISSN

Gimpel, T.: Therapy by colour, Brook House, Tetbury, England 80

Giudice,E.del: Coherence in condensed and living matter, Frontier Perspectives, Vol. 3, No. 2, 16-20, 1993. (This applies, among other things, to the options for storing of EM signals)

Guidice E.

del, Elia V.:     Role of water in living organisms. Neurale Network

Goernitz, Th.:  Quanta are different, Spektrum 2011

The creative cosmos, Springer Spectrum 2013

Light, quanta and consciousness

From quanta to consciousness, 2016

Grossarth-      Autonomy training; „Disease as Biography", KiWi

Maticek, R.:    Synergistic Prevention Medicine, Springer 2008

Hager, E. D.:   Complementary Oncology, Forum Medizin- Publisher

Society 1997

Hartenbach:     The cholesterol lie, Weltbild- Publisher

Heim, B.:       The elementary process of life, Resch Innsbruck 94

Elementary structures of matter. Resch Innsbruck 1985

The cosmic human experience space, Resch 1995

Post-mortem conditions? The tele variant area of

integral world structures, Resch- Publisher 1994

Uniform description of the material world, 1994

Hildebrandt:    Circadian rhythms as the basis of a therapeutic time

order, ÄZN 8/87, 27. Year 1987

Hauf, R.:       Influence of electromagnetic fields on humans,

etz-b, 28, 181-183, 1976

Heber, G..      Introduction to the theory of magnetism, Wissensch.

Buchgesellschaft Darmstadt 1983

Heine, H.:      Reduction of radicals in the basic substance through

polysaccharide-silica-water complexes" Ärztezeitschrift

für NHV 12/03, 897-902

Textbook of the biological medicine" Hippokrates

Publisher 1991

Superordinate regulatory principles of the extracellular

basic substance (matrix) for prophylaxis and regene-

ration, Schweiz. Zeitschrift f. Ganzheitsmedizin 2/89,

Heine, H.: Disorders – Chronic Illness – Aging, CO.med-Edition 2009

Heiß,G.Hrsg.: Cancer…what now? Perspectives of the 21. Century Darmstadt, Merz Publisher 2001

Hoffmann, M.

Wolf, G.,

Staller, B.: Redox potentials in food and their health relevance for environmental medicine in No. 33, edition 2/00

Hoffmann,M: Food Quality – Quality of Life, a holistic view, Ganz-heitsmedizin 1 (1987) 12

Three-dimensional quality test in field vegetable growing, in Heilmann, H., Zimmer, U. (Editor): Alternative Concepts No 72 Karlsruhe 1990

Food quality & health, baeren & fuss

Food & nutrition from an electrochemical point of view, CO.med 05/05

Karstaedt, U.: The acid of life, TAS- Publisher London

Karsten, H.: Fragrance-color-tone therapy for psychosomatic Illnesses, Haug Publisher 1983

Kiene, H.: Complementary medicine-conventional medicine. Science dispute at the end of the 20th century, 2nd edition 1996

Koehler, B.: See page 134-135

Synergistic biological cancer treatment, CO'MED edition 1998

Symmetropathy, integration by communication

Koenig, M.: The origin word, The physics of GOD, Scorpio 2010

Kremer, H.: Cancer and AIDS medicine, ZDN 2001

Krueger, W.: The eye of the needle for colors and tones, Atom Harmonik Publisher

Lamy, J. in: Organism and tone, Schick, E.

Langreder,W:  From the biological to biophysical medicine,
              Haug Publisher 1985
Laszlo, E.:   Coherence in cosmos and consciousness, Via Nova
              Publisher 2003
Lipton, B.:   Intelligent cells, 3.Auflage, KOHA- Publisher 2007
Ludwig, W.:   Oscillation therapy. Naturheilpraxis 32, 1026-1030
              New electromagnetic diagnose and therapy methods,
              Bulletin ASE/UCS 80, 928-932 (1979)
              SIT System Information Therapy, Spitta- Publisher 94
              Informative Medicine, VGM- Publisher 1998
              The expanded unified quantum field theory of Burkhard
              Heim, Resch Publisher 1998
Luescher, M.: The regulation psychology of colours, Lehr-CD
              The harmonic law in us, Ullstein Publisher Berlin
              The 4 colour man, Ullstein Publisher 2009
Lutz, W.:     Living without bread, 16. Auflage, Informed GmbH, 07
Meyl, K.:     Electromagnetic environmental compatibility, Band
              1+2, Indel Publisher VS 1996
              Potential vortexes, volume I & II, Indel Publi. VS 1990
Mercola, J.:  EMF, Electromagnetic Fields, Kopp Publisher 2020
Muheim,J.T.:  On the universal role of elementary particles. Rapport
              de la Réunion de printemps de la Société Suisse des
              Physique 56, 925-928 (1983)
Mueller, G.:  viva vortex, all lives, BOD 2016
Mutter, J.:   Healthy instead of chronically ill, fit for life Publisher
              Do not be poisoned, Gräfe & Unser Publisher
Ohlenschl.C.: The interactions between light and biomolecules, EHK
              5/91, Volume 40
Pauli, W.:    The general principles of wave mechanics, Springer
Penrose, R:   Shadow of the Mind, Path to a New Physics of Consci-
              ousness, Spectrum Academic Publishing House (1995)

Peseschkian:      Positive psychotherapy; Believe in God and fix your camel, Herder Publisher

Pischinger,A:     The system of basic regulation, Haug-Publisher 1989

Plichta, P.:      The prime number cross, volume 1-5 Quadropol-Publisher 2000

Pokorný J.:       Froehlichs coherent vibrations in healthy and cancer cells. Neural Network World Vol.19, Nr 4, 369-378, 09

Pollack,G.H.:     The 4. phase of water, VAK Publischer

Popp, F. A.:      Biophotones. Verlag f. Medizin, Publ. Dr. E. Fischer, Electromagnetic Bio-Information. Urban&Schwarzenberg-Publisher 1989

Popp, F. A.,
Strauss,V.E.:     Molecular and biophysical aspects of malignity. Praxis Publisher, Leer 1984

Presman,A.S.:     Electromagnetic fields and life, Plenum Press 1970

Priebe, L.:       Vegetative, Rhythm, Chaos. ÄZN 6/1989, 30. year. Medicine and deterministic chaos, EHK 1/90

Risi, A.:         You are life beings, Gorinda Publisher
                  The radical middle ground, Kopp Publisher 2009

Rosenberg:        Solving conflicts through nonviolent communication, 15. edition, Herder Publisher 2012

Rubbia, C.:       Nobel award 1984 for the experimental proof of the interaction quanta superordinate to matter, which control the structure of matter.

Russel, W.:       Secret of light, Genius Publisher 2002
                  Radioactivity, the death principle of nature, Genius

Schick, E.:       Organism and tone, Hirschberger Publisher 1987

Schmidt/Peters Microbiologic Therapy, AMT 2004

Schole/Lutz:      Regulation diseases, 2. edition BoD 2001

Schroedinger:     What is life?

Schumann,W: About the radiation less natural vibrations of a conductive sphere surrounded by a layer of air and an ionospheric shell. Zeitschrift für Naturforschung 7a, 149-154, 1954

Selby, J.:   Breathing naturally, holistic health by breath-Integration Sphinx Publisher Basel 1984

Selye, H.:   Introduction to the teaching of adapter systems, G. Thieme Publisher, Stuttgart 1953

Sheldrake,R.: The creating universe, Meyster Publisher, Munich 1983
The Presence of the Past, Times book
The memory of the nature, Scherz Publisher 1990

Smith,C.W.:   Electromagnetic Phenomena in Living Biomedical Systems, Proc.6, Anual Conf. IEEE 1984

Spalinger, K.: Death: happy, life without limited thinking, Hagal-Publisher 1997

Temelie, B.:   Nutrition according to the 5 elements, Joy Publisher Sulzberg

Trincher, K.:   Nature and spirit, Herder Publisher, Wien 1981
The laws of the biological thermodynamic, Urban & Schwarzenberg Publisher, Wien 1981
Water. Basic structure of life and thought, Herder Wien

Voeikov, V:   Fundamental role of water in bioenergetics. In: Belousov L, Voeikov V, Martynyuk V: Biophotonics and coherent systems in biology, Springer Publisher 07

Warnke, U.:   Human and the third force, Popular Academic Publisher, Saarbrücken 1994

Wever, R.:   ELF-effects on human circadian rhythm, In: Persinger,
M.A.:   ELF and VLF electromagnetic field effects, Plenum

Wilber, K.:   The holographic worldview, Scherz Publisher

Worm, N.:   Human foie gras, systemed Publisher
Common disease fatty liver, systemed Publisher

Zabel, W.:    Nutrition and Cancer, lecture on ZÄN-Congress

Zeiger, B.:    Information medicine & cosmology, www.bit-org.de

Zoech, W.:    Embryonic origin of carcinoma, lecture on Medicine Week Baden-Baden 2015

# *Sources*

www.bit-org.de     International medical society for **B**iophysical **I**nformation **T**herapy **BIT** e.V. (LSIT)

www.solumed.eu     Source of supply for the high quality dietary supplements **KlinSiMag®**, **CurSiMag®**, **Glukosa-K2®** (all vegan) and **Neptune NKO Krill-Oil**

www.sdg-vertrieb.de Source of supply for the **Equalizer EQ 103** and the new **LYMPHO*DYN*®** device and books

www.apodil.de     Nosodes and organ preparations

**Note:** ZMR 703, Vortex 705, NEC 708 and MRT 503 are no longer in production and are only on the market as used devices.

A selection of holistic biological clinics in Germany:

Klink St. Georg, 83043 Bad Aibling, Rosenheimer Straße 6
phone 08061 3980, Internet www.klinik-st-georg.de

Biomed-Klinik 76887 Bad Bergzabern, Tischbergerstraße 5
phone 06343 7050, Internet www.biomedklinik.de

Klinik im Leben 07973 Greiz, Gartenweg 5-6
phone 03661 4438210, Internet www.klinik-imleben.de